CU00869565

Louise Roddon is a respected journalist specialising in health and lifestyle topics. Her articles have appeared in *The Times*, the *Daily Mail*, *Today*, the *Evening Standard* and the *European* as well as many leading magazines.

She has changed from being a keen fan of good wine, rich foods, cigarettes and a lazy lifestyle to someone who now exercises regularly, eats properly, sleeps well and still has a great sense of humour!

Jacky Fleming is a best-selling cartoonist. Her books, *Be a Bloody Train Driver*, *Never Give Up* and *Falling in Love* are published by Penguin.

AM I A MONSTER, OR IS THIS PMS?

Self help for PMS sufferers

Louise Roddon

HEADLINE

First published in 1994
by HEADLINE BOOK PUBLISHING

10 9 8 7 6 5 4 3 2 1

ISBN 0 7472 4337 9

Typeset by
Letterpart Limited, Reigate, Surrey

Printed and bound in Great Britain by
HarperCollins Manufacturing, Glasgow

HEADLINE BOOK PUBLISHING
A division of Hodder Headline PLC
Headline House
79 Great Titchfield Street
London W1P 7FN

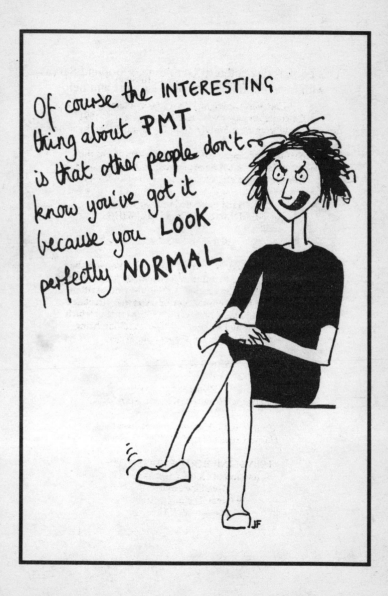

This book is dedicated to Geraldine, Flora and Sarah
with love and thanks for their support and help

Contents

CHAPTER 1

PMS – Fact or Fantasy?

MAGGIE'S STORY

Maggie sat stirring her cappuccino and confessed to me just how miserable she felt.

'I can't seem to do a thing right,' she sighed. 'I fly off the handle at the slightest thing; I bitch at the kids, and if Ian tries to show me any sympathy, I bite his head off. Sometimes I just want to pick a fight with him to release all this tension. I'm like a monster in my own home. I just don't recognise myself. It never used to be like this. When I was at school, the only indication I had that my period was due was a dull ache in my stomach – and that was that. The older I get, the worse my symptoms become.

'On top of the irritability, I get very tearful and I suffer from blinding headaches. And to make matters worse, I seem to put on a hell of a lot of weight. My clothes don't fit for at least a fortnight. My stomach feels swollen and bloated, and my breasts are horrifically tender. Oh, and I get spots, too – God, it's great being a woman.'

If Maggie's story rings any bells, the chances are that you are one of the many justifiably miserable women who suffers from premenstrual syndrome. Like Maggie, you may have despaired of ever finding relief for your symptoms. Perhaps your doctor is unsympathetic; maybe s/he has prescribed an anti-depressant which you don't feel like taking, or possibly, faced with a lack of sympathy, you are beginning to believe you have imagined these symptoms, and that the shattering black hole you slip into each month is actually part of your temperament.

Like Maggie, too, you may be totally confused by the range of heavily marketed over-the-counter remedies now on sale in chemists. Should you try that expensive Evening Primrose Oil – or the new Starflower Oil? Will vitamins do the job just as well? Or should you just bury your head in the sand, write a dozen letters of apology to your nearest and dearest, and hive off to the nearest desert island?

Rest assured there is sensible and easy-to-follow help at hand for the sufferer. And there is a safe path through the fashions in 'designer' remedies. Remember, whether your symptoms are chronically severe, or merely annoyingly 'regular', PMS is a very real condition, and there are billions of bad-tempered and bloated women throughout the world who, just like you, probably fear they are exaggerating their symptoms. Whatever the sceptical might think, this vastly united front just goes to prove that we can't all be lying!

MY STORY

Like my friend Maggie, my premenstrual symptoms have become more extreme over the years. At school, I just put up with abdominal cramps at the onset of my period; indeed, I almost welcomed them, because at least I had a good excuse to get out of hockey practice!

My worst symptoms spanned depression, despair and tearfulness on the psychological side; and on the physical, tender breasts, water retention, clumsiness (you could guarantee I would break something just before my period) and spots.

Now I know people claim that they alone have the best cure, and that's the one you should try, ignoring all others – but since writing this book, I have enjoyed a life free of these irritating monthly symptoms. If anything, it comes as a complete surprise to me when my period arrives. My breasts no longer swell or get sore; the water retention is vastly reduced, the depression and despair have lessened – and the nasty adolescent-style spots have gone. It's like going back to my schooldays!

Obviously over a period of time I tried as many as I could of the suggestions given in this book. What seems to work best for me is a combination of the low-fat, high-carbohydrate diet recommended in Chapter 14, together with regular exercise, a mineral and vitamin supplement and a conscious aim on my part to allow for an hour of total relaxation each day. I've cut my manic coffee consumption down to a maximum of two cups a day, taken in the morning (it was easier than I dared imagine) and I drink lots of water. I feel fitter, younger, healthier and less scratchy! Homeopathic remedies have also played a part in my relief from PMS and these I describe in Chapter 11.

My best advice to you, if you have consulted your GP and you truly suffer from PMS, is to decide for yourself which of the many suggestions I give will fit happily into your own particular lifestyle – and having made your decision, try sticking to that chosen regime for at least three months, so that you can gauge the effectiveness of the remedies. Go on, you've nothing to lose – and the chances are you will feel a lot healthier for it!

WHAT IS PMS?

A seemingly daft question, this, especially if you are a sufferer. But even those lucky women who don't suffer any misery before their periods will undoubtedly know that PMS stands for premenstrual syndrome.

Amazingly enough, there still exists a large percentage of men who have no idea what these three power-packed letters mean, nor even what PMT, the original and less broad-ranging term, stands for.

Women tend to be very clued up on the subject and assume everyone else is – so much so that a female employee of the BBC recently joked to me how in her early days at Broadcasting House, she noticed there was a special PMT room.

'I thought what considerate employers the Beeb were – and then I noticed that men kept on going into that room. Of course I soon learnt that PMT also stands for "photomechanical transfer" . . .'

There have been nearly as many theories about the causes of premenstrual syndrome as there are symptoms. Probably no individual theory embraces the whole truth, though there is truth in many of them. PMS is the umbrella term for a number of physical and psychological symptoms which can happen at any time during the two to fourteen days before menstruation. These symptoms usually disappear completely at the onset of bleeding.

Menstruation always did have a scabby reputation – what with curdling milk and blighting crops, but it took twentieth-century science to discover that women could be possessed by nasty spirits *before* their periods had even begun. In 1931, a certain Dr R.H.T. Frank published a psychiatric paper in which he described a handful of women who suffered from what he termed 'premenstrual tension' – a time of stress and hostility for women. The more recent term PMS refers to more wide-ranging symptoms; if, for example, you experience fluid retention, headaches, depression and tender breasts, then you are probably a PMS sufferer.

Today, few women challenge the fact that PMS is a condition which affects the whole body, though recently a group of psychologists did exactly that. 'All in the mind' was their scathing verdict on the syndrome – but more on the sceptics and their reasonings in Chapter 23.

Dr Katharina Dalton, former chiropodist and now Britain's leading PMS expert who first used the phrase PMS in 1953, cites some 150 recognisable symptoms. She discovered that while PMS sufferers seem to function well physically for part of each month, during the PMS phase it is as if the body's signals are crossed or distorted, both physically and psychologically. So – before you think you are going completely mad, rest assured that if that irritability, bloated belly, clumsiness and tearfulness occur *only cyclically*, then you are not the

4

grumpy monster with a foul personality that you probably believe yourself to be.

The figures

My story and Maggie's are by no means typical. Symptoms do vary from sufferer to sufferer, and here are some figures to help reassure you that you are certainly not alone in your monthly misery:

★ 95% of women in Britain experience PMS symptoms
★ 25% of teenagers in Europe suffer from PMS
★ 50% of adult women suffer PMS severely enough to cause significant disruption to their lives
★ 30% of women who shoplift are premenstrual
(source: Dr Katharina Dalton)

PMS IN HISTORY

If PMS had been discovered centuries ago, rather than relatively recently in 1931, the course of history might have taken a very different path. Indeed, if you examine some of the female 'greats' from the past, and adjust your thinking to take in the idea that they too might have suffered from PMS, then history could almost be re-written under the new, more appropriate heading of 'Her Story'. There's every chance that Cleopatra, Catherine the Great, Lady Macbeth, and those seventeenth-century 'witches' burnt at the stake all suffered from the syndrome – even the Empress Josephine could be among them. If she, like other women, felt put off sex during her premenstrual phase, there should perhaps be a new question mark on the end of Napoleon's famous line: 'Not tonight, Josephine'.

Until the nineteenth century, doctors believed that the womb was the seat of all women's troubles. For centuries, it was thought that the womb moved around the body, causing all sorts of ills, and making women behave in the most peculiar

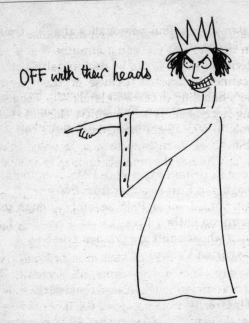

OFF with their heads

manner. If this were true, it would be quite understandable for women to feel moody!

Once hormones were 'discovered' at the beginning of this century, they took the starring role as the cause for women's unpredictability. The 'raging hormone theory', as it was known, stated that women were hapless victims of their hormones, from which there was no escape. Such a belief was often used as an excuse for not letting women take responsible jobs – an excuse amazingly sustained even as recently as 1970. Karen Paige, a psychologist who has studied premenstrual mood changes, quotes an American doctor from that year who said: 'If you had an investment in a bank, you wouldn't want the president of the bank making a loan under those raging hormonal influences at that particular period. Suppose we had a president in the White House, a menopausal woman president, who had to make the decision of the Bay of Pigs, which was, of course, a bad one, or about the Russian contretemps with Cuba at that time?'

6

That 'woman president' might well have made a good decision, given the job. But you can guarantee that if she had made a bad decision, there would be doctors telling the world that women cannot be trusted because of 'their hormones'. Even Thatcher's handling of the Falklands War has been put down to raging hormones by the sceptics. Hormonal change does have a role to play in the menstrual cycle, but it is not certain whether these hormonal swings actually cause the mood changes, or whether they merely happen to coincide with them.

Though not recognised as a condition until the thirties, PMS has most certainly been around for a very long time. Virginia Woolf, the British novelist, expressed what have to be PMS symptoms very succinctly in a diary entry for 1928:

'I had thought to write the quickest most brilliant pages in *Orlando* yesterday – not a drop came, all, forsooth, for the usual physical reasons, which delivered themselves today. It is the oddest feeling: as if a finger stopped the flow of ideas in the brain; it is unsealed and the blood rushes all over the place.'

Sounds familiar? Apathy, sluggishness, and a feeling of ineptitude are common symptoms of PMS – of which more later.

Certainly, premenstrual symptoms have been experienced and observed for centuries, but acknowledging them as a real condition, and treating them with understanding, is a relatively recent phenomenon.

CHAPTER 2

Cutting Through the Crossed Wires

(Thank God, it's Only My Period!)

How often have you uttered those thanks on the first day of bleeding, or heard them from the lips of a friend? One of the baffling aspects of PMS is that sufferers tend to forget they are undergoing this nasty cyclical change in character, and believe they are really ill – or turning into monsters. This belief in itself illustrates not only how powerful the symptoms can be, but also how those crossed signals or wires that Dr Dalton talks about can operate on every conscious level. We lose our grip on reality. Balance flies out of the window. 'I'm going mad,' we cry. 'I've got flu!' – 'I've put on weight, even though I haven't pigged out on muffins!' – 'My marriage/career/children are a disaster!' Only at the last possible moment do we do a mental calendar check – sometimes waiting until the first sighting of blood – before looking at the possibility that PMS may be at work.

As Vanessa, aged twenty-seven, says: 'I never think my tearfulness or grumpiness is due to PMS. I go around raging and making my husband's life a misery. When my period starts, it's such a relief that one day I said to him: "Can't you remind me that it's just PMS?" Well, the next month he did just that, and I practically bit his head off: "How *dare* you say I'm premenstrual!" Poor guy, he can't win!'

So what are these 'crossed wires' – and why do some women suffer more acutely than others?

The general belief is that the body has a control centre in the brain known as the hypothalamus. This is located in the part

8

of the brain where the nerve and hormonal systems are integrated. The hypothalamus receives nerve and hormonal messages as well as sending out messages which control the body's functions. The crossed-wire syndrome could well be explained as the hypothalamus, or 'conductor', going awry during part of each menstrual cycle.

WHAT DOES THIS CONDUCTOR DO?

The hypothalamus is connected to the parts of the nervous system which affect heart rate, blood pressure, muscular movement in the intestines and stomach, and heat regulation. It is also involved in the production of hormones affecting the breasts, thyroid gland, adrenal glands, ovaries, kidneys (affecting the balance of body fluids), blood (changing the blood sugar level) and uterus (causing contractions and starting labour).

More specifically, the hypothalamus controls certain functions which some experts believe operate poorly during the premenstrual phase. These include a weight control centre to regulate body weight; emotional centres for the control of emotions such as anxiety, fear and rage; and an appetite centre which registers hunger and satisfaction, so influencing eating behaviour. If you've ever wondered why you periodically get the urge to binge on biscuits, you can now excuse your weakness as being down to those 'crossed wires' – and not necessarily a case of greed doing battle with self-control!

Many of these 'centres' have definite links with common PMS symptoms: bingeing, water retention, dizziness, tender breasts, not to mention rage and depression – yet why the hypothalamus should go awry cyclically is not fully understood.

OTHER PHYSICAL THEORIES

It may well be true that certain women suffering a hormonal

imbalance are more prone to PMS, but it is not necessarily correct to say that all cases are related to hormones. Unfortunately, some doctors are rather dismissive of patients with PMS and tend to turn to hormonal theories and treatments as a ready remedy for chronic cases. Generally, I would stress that you look into these treatments only after trying out some of the many self-help suggestions given in the following chapters.

However, it is certainly advisable to consult your GP if you are suffering from PMS. Many doctors are very knowledgeable on the subject and they may help you with diet and with finding the best contraceptive to suit your symptoms. Also, it is as well to check that it is PMS which is really affecting you.

An imbalance of oestrogen and progesterone

This theory was first suggested by Dr Katharina Dalton, who made a distinction between spasmodic and congestive dysmenorrhoea. Congestive pain is nagging, accompanied by lethargy and water retention – a characteristic of PMS for many women. Spasmodic pain is sharp and cramping – usually associated with the bleeding itself. Dr Dalton's belief is that congestive pain results from too little progesterone in the second half of the cycle; spasmodic, from too little oestrogen. Progesterone injections or pessaries have certainly helped a number of sufferers to find relief (see Chapter 5) and in one study conducted at a London hospital, progesterone was found to relieve distress in about 30% of cases. However, a survey conducted by the Women's Nutritional Advisory Service reveals that progesterone pessaries have shown no benefit when compared with a placebo – and that they have no place in the treatment of PMS.

Prolactin

Some researchers have found a link between raised prolactin levels (prolactin is a hormone produced by the pituitary gland which affects the breasts and ovaries; its chief role is in stimulating milk production) and breast symptoms in women.

Prolactin is also known to affect water and mineral balances, and this has led some doctors to suggest that the hormone plays a part in the sore breast/water retention symptoms of PMS. A number of doctors have tried a new drug out on patients which lowers the amount of prolactin in the blood during the second half of the cycle, and it seems to make some women feel less bloated.

Vitamin and mineral deficiency
A fair amount of research has been conducted into the link between vitamin and mineral deficiency and PMS. I will discuss these in Chapter 9.

PSYCHOLOGICAL THEORIES – SOME OF THE REASONS WHY YOU FEEL LIKE A GRUMPY MONSTER

Mental illness does not cause PMS; you can be emotionally disturbed with or without PMS. And at the same time, emotionally healthy, outgoing women are still prone to the syndrome. In other words, you will be relieved to learn that your essential personality does not necessarily predispose you towards suffering from PMS. However, if you are going through an emotional crisis *unrelated* to PMS, then the chances are you will suffer the symptoms of PMS more acutely during that period.

'I must try my best'
Interestingly, there is thought to be a link between perfectionism and PMS. If you are the sort of sufferer who tries to maintain very high standards of behaviour and control in work, in relationships and in your emotional life, then it is likely you will be more easily shaken than others when you find yourself unable to meet those high standards. This is not to say that PMS is more common among perfectionists – but the effect of some symptoms is likely to be greater.

CHAPTER 3

The Many Faces of PMS

If you are a sufferer, you probably don't need to be told what the symptoms of PMS are – but you may not be familiar with all of them. Very few women at any one given time suffer anywhere near the total of 150 symptoms thought to be linked to PMS, and it is also true to say that some sufferers experience their symptoms more acutely than others. And, of course, the symptoms themselves may vary from month to month.

It may also come as some surprise to you to learn, for example, that dry, itchy eyes are linked to PMS – perhaps, if you wear them, you had mistakenly thought you needed to change your contact lenses; likewise, not every woman realises that PMS can make her more sensitive to alcohol. If you recently went through one of those awful late-night rows with your husband or partner, and the next morning you can't remember what started it – or indeed what was said – think how much you had to drink the night before and, if it was no more than your usual intake, a check with your calendar may help to link your overreactive rowing session to a date within your premenstrual phase. If not – well, that's another matter altogether, and perhaps your 'normal' alcohol intake is veering towards the abnormal!

As varied as these symptoms are, the common link is that they are experienced cyclically as opposed to all the time – and thank goodness for that! Generally, they occur some time after ovulation and end with menstruation.

CHARACTERISTICS OF PMS SYMPTOMS

★ They can range from mild to severe – and sufferers can experience both mild symptoms and severe ones during any given year.

★ They can last from one or two days to two weeks. Some sufferers can experience symptoms during the beginning of menstruation too. A recent survey undertaken by the support group PMS Help showed that women suffered an average of thirteen symptoms: the core complaints being irritability, tension, sore breasts and headaches.

★ PMS symptoms can occur at any point in a woman's life, from her first menstrual period, to after a hysterectomy, and through into menopause.

★ Age can and often does increase the severity of symptoms.

★ Childbirth, too, can increase severity.

★ They can occur after a trauma, either physical or mental.

★ They can occur some months, and not others.

★ The symptoms usually disappear each month at the onset of bleeding or soon after it occurs.

★ One in three women have to take time off work because PMS has made them feel so bad; half of them will lie about why they are absent, as they are too embarrassed to tell the truth.

Let's look first at some of the most common symptoms of PMS, how they manifest themselves, and what causes them.

PHYSICAL SYMPTOMS

Fluid retention: beating the bulging tum
Picture this all-too-familiar scenario: you've got an important evening function to attend. You know the other women attending will all be Lycra-clad lovelies, so only that chic, black and terribly tight cocktail dress will do (Laura Ashley floral is definitely a no-no). You've been dieting to look your best, but on the morning of the important day you wake up with a

bulging, bloated tum, big enough to have everyone thinking you are five months pregnant.

This has to be one of the worst of the most common symptoms, simply because of its psychological effects on the sufferer and because it seems all too visibly apparent – at least, to the sufferer. And when your self-esteem is likely to be at an all-time rock bottom anyway – especially if you've just behaved like a cow to your nearest and dearest – a bloated belly can indeed seem like the last straw. It's there as a constant reminder. You sit down and folds of unsightly flesh concertina in your lap; stand up, and your profile reveals an unwanted spare tyre. Forget the slinky black dress; only a sack dress will cover this lot!

Fluid retention is the bane of PMS sufferers. It occurs because, premenstrually, water collects in the tissues of the abdomen (and sometimes in the ankles and face too) as the body fluids are being redistributed. For some women, fluid

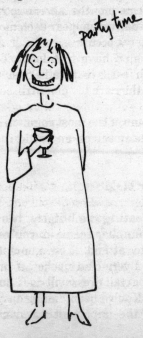

retention can be so severe that they can gain around ten to twelve extra pounds in weight; even their shoes feel tight, and their eyes, too, may look puffy. For these women, a complete set of different-sized clothes has often been the only answer, though most women only gain an extra three to four pounds in weight. But whatever the amount, water retention is likely to make you feel extremely touchy, introverted and self-conscious.

WHY DOES FLUID RETENTION OCCUR?
The premenstrual sufferer is experiencing an excess of the hormone aldosterone. This hormone is produced by the adrenal glands, which are found just above the kidneys. The adrenal glands control the kidneys' water and salt retention. When balanced, aldosterone is an essential hormone, but when produced in excess (usually because oestrogen levels are too high), it can cause the body to retain water and salt – hence that unsightly bloating. Bloatedness may also be associated with a lack of calcium, or with a temporary pyridoxine (vitamin B6) deficiency. A change of diet (foods rich in vitamin B6 include brown rice, walnuts, almonds, liver, avocado pears.) can really help, as can calcium-rich foods. Topping up on these vitamins, whether in pill format or in food, for ten days before a period can do wonders, not only with bloating but equally with headaches and general abdominal pain. As we will see in the following chapters, dietary changes can be a tremendous asset in relieving many symptoms of PMS.

Sore breasts
'When I take off my bra at night, it's like letting go of a heavy shopping bag – my breasts seem to spill out. They feel hot to the touch, and my bra cuts uncomfortably into them. I can't bear having my breasts touched at this point. When the cat jumps on top of me, I nearly scream out in pain, and if Ian tries to fondle my nipples, I have a terrible urge to hit him. As soon as my period starts, they return to normal size – and this is enough to cheer me up out of all proportion.' (Maggie, aged thirty-six.)

Maggie suffers from sore breasts premenstrually, far more

acutely than from any of the other common physical symptoms. Breast tenderness is a very common premenstrual symptom, and ranges in characteristics from general swelling, lumpiness around the outside of the breast and even near the underarm, to sharp pain experienced down the arm – usually more extreme in the morning and at night. Breast cysts, if they exist, can become enlarged at this time, and even women with smooth tissue may experience mastitis (lumpiness).

An excess of prolactin (see Chapter 2) is often responsible for breast swelling. There are anti-prolactin drugs on the market which inhibit the hormone, but bromocriptine, to give this drug its correct name, is a powerful chemical to take into a healthy body. In large doses, it can cause nausea and vomiting – hardly a welcome addition to your other PMS symptoms. More pertinently, given that prolactin tends to inhibit ovulation, if you take a drug which inhibits this hormone, you can increase your chances of becoming pregnant.

One breast cancer specialist I know swears by Evening Primrose Oil, which he also sees as especially helpful for PMS sufferers. The benefits of Evening Primrose Oil are discussed in Chapter 9.

Headaches and lethargy

'I feel like a slug,' says Susan, a normally active twenty-five-year-old. 'I don't want to do anything except crawl under the duvet. The slightest movement makes my head bang, I can't be bothered to cook, and I have no enthusiasm for anything.'

Lethargy, usually accompanied by headaches and sugar craving, is a typical PMS symptom. For normally active women, these symptoms can be very debilitating; for those with a depressive tendency, increased lethargy during the premenstrual phase can seem particularly traumatic.

Geraldine, aged forty, confesses to a terrible sweet tooth during her premenstrual phase – a symptom shared by 68% of sufferers in a recent survey.

'It quite shocks me. It's as if I'm a zombie. Sometimes I look at my car after I've had a binge, and it's full of sweetie wrappings and empty chocolate foil. I can barely remember eating them, and when I see how much I have eaten, well, that just makes me feel worse – really irritable and even more aggressive.'

The reason that I have coupled these symptoms together – lethargy, headache and sugar craving – is that they tend to be interrelated. And these symptoms, because they challenge one's idea of self-control – i.e., the desire to conquer those depressing female evils of laziness and binge-eating – can trigger the emotional PMS symptoms of depression, irritability, self-loathing and tearfulness.

Women who crave sugar often experience headaches, heart pounding and fatigue – and sometimes dizziness. This is due to swings in blood sugar levels, and, likewise, PMS headache sufferers are usually women who take in too much caffeine. Satisfying the craving for sweet foods and chocolate usually sets up a vicious circle of headaches, lethargy and dizziness; when energy levels fall, symptoms of nervousness may occur.

For women with eating disorders, the 'crossed wires' of PMS can exacerbate these disorders. Bingers tend to binge more during the premenstrual phase, while anorexics are likely to starve themselves more actively during this phase, in anticipation of cravings and weight gain through fluid retention. Again, a wholesome change in diet may well help, which is outlined in Chapters 13 and 14.

Smell sensitivity

Seemingly an obscure one, this, but it is surprising how many women admit to having a heightened sense of smell during their premenstrual phase.

'It's very odd,' says thirty-five-year-old Helen, 'but I can smell the oddest of smells before my period – not always nice ones, either. It took me a long time to work out that it had anything to do with PMS. But I was doing a project on health for work and I kept a PMS diary for a couple of months and that's when it became obvious that there was a link between these smells and my cycle.

'I smell odd stuff like babies' gripe water, candy floss, new-mown grass, and, most difficult of all, burning. I'm constantly looking into waste-paper baskets to see if they're on fire. At work, I might suddenly say, 'Ooh, I can smell candy floss.' The girls in the office have got quite used to this, and usually tell me my period is due – sometimes it's my only gauge that it is "that time of the month". Sure enough, one or two days later, my period will start. At the same time, I become extremely clumsy. I know that I'm more likely to drop a cigarette because my spatial judgement has gone, and then I will often smell burning. It's enough to make me very paranoid.'

A sensitivity to smells – not necessarily accurate, either – is linked also to a sensitivity to noise, light and touch. Some women find the television or radio unbearably loud at this time, to the point that it will almost reduce them to tears. Babies crying can be another irritant – and touch, too, can seem unbearable. I know of one woman who can't stand wearing wool at this time; another complains that her jewellery irritates. It's all part of the crossed wires syndrome. In some ways, PMS resembles a heightened state of consciousness – almost like being in a different world and looking at life through a magnifying glass. If you think about these heightened senses – the heightened craving for sweet things, the relief you feel once you've emerged from a black cloud – that heightened sense of consciousness soon becomes evident. One school of thought is that if you rejoice in that heightened state of consciousness – in the sense of actively welcoming the feeling of being alive to your surroundings – then this positive attitude can itself alleviate symptoms. Thinking negatively about menstruation, as in a way we have been conditioned to do (the very word 'curse' says it all), will only exacerbate the pain and related symptoms of menstruation.

Again, a hormonal imbalance – an abnormal level of endorphins – goes some way to explaining these heightened sensations. Think of how pregnant women find that things taste very differently from normal; the same in a sense applies to the PMS sufferer. Relaxation techniques (see Chapters 6 and 7) and

Evening Primrose Oil can be of great benefit to these symptoms.

Clumsiness, lack of coordination

'I always know when my period is coming, because without fail I'll drop something. I usually break a mug or glass at this time.' (Laura, aged twenty-eight.)

A lot of women complain they feel clumsy at this time. It is often a physical manifestation of other typical psychological PMS symptoms: confusion and absent-mindedness. You know that feeling of spaciness – of not quite being there, of feeling dithery? Many women forget what they were about to say or do, and this can be a very distressing state, especially if you are in a high-powered job where you need to be on the ball. Some women find this state to be so incapacitating that it adversely affects their work; for others, exercise can be of real benefit.

The cause of premenstrual clumsiness is difficult to fathom. It may be due to a disturbance in the finer aspects of the nervous system, occurring premenstrually. This can be caused by changes in brain chemistry, hormonal chemistry, an excessive intake of coffee, tea, cigarettes or alcohol, or a deficiency in certain nutrients.

Other physical symptoms
abdominal cramps
acne
alcohol intolerance
back pain
constipation, followed by diarrhoea
eye problems
haemorrhoids
hand tingling and numbness
herpes
insomnia
muscle ache
sex-drive changes
urinary difficulties

CHAPTER 4

Psychological Symptoms

Probably the most distressing factor of PMS is the extent to which the syndrome can affect us psychologically. Some women complain of feeling completely off the wall; others experience acute personality changes; and even for the majority of sufferers who labour under a black cloud of temporary irritability and depression, life can seem very bleak indeed. It is the emotional symptoms above all others which are likely to inspire a woman to come forward for help with PMS. Women tend to be more worried about the effects of their PMS on their families, friends and colleagues than on themselves.

As I indicated in the first chapter, the first step in learning to deal with PMS is to accept that you *will* change for a period of time and to encourage those closest to realise and accept this too. This sounds easy, but it can prove quite a difficult task. None of us wants to appear moody and unpredictable – mothers and lovers are looked to for dependability and strength – and, surprisingly, there is still a stigma surrounding any talk of periods, so casually mentioning you are suffering from PMS doesn't always pay off. It may work at home; indeed, many understanding partners can be very helpful in predicting when your period is likely to start, given the evidence of your change in mood – especially if you're in that cycle where PMS is the last condition you would attach to this temporary mad state. The chapters dedicated to partners may be of help here. Even so, office colleagues, especially male colleagues, may not always prove to be so understanding. Given the struggle women have had to gain acceptance in the workforce, a cynical male colleague is likely to react unfavourably if you explain away your short-temperedness as 'merely my PMS'.

Self-help health groups and women's groups (see Chapter 22) can be of enormous help in learning to understand and cope with these changes in mood: again, the importance of talking about how you feel cannot be overstressed. If it seems too sensitive to raise these issues at home, the chance to 'share' your experiences with like-minded females and to gain some insight into how they cope themselves, can prove a tremendous relief and aid. Some women have even found that the more they talk about their symptoms in a positive way, the less distressing their PMS becomes.

If your PMS consists mostly of psychological symptoms – ranging from anxiety and irritability to depression, tearfulness and palpitations, your doctor may well prescribe a tranquilliser or anti-depressant. These, if possible, should be avoided. Tranquillisers are now known to be addictive, never mind the dopey-making side-effects associated with their use. If you find it hard to cope with simple tasks while suffering from PMS, then this aspect of the drug will only heighten the sensation that you are functioning less efficiently than normal.

Similarly, some women suffer premenstrual anxiety more acutely during some months than others. If this is the case, it may be worth examining what is going on in your life to cause that anxiety. This is not to discount anxiety as a genuine psychological symptom of PMS but to indicate that like all PMS symptoms the functions of the body, whether physical or psychological, get heightened during this period. You may be suffering from a stress overload during certain months and PMS is likely to exacerbate this stress. Try looking at the root cause of the stress rather than resorting to tranquillisers.

Likewise, anti-depressants won't necessarily help to cure the cyclical depression that occurs as part of PMS, since the majority of the anti-depressants that doctors prescribe take at least two weeks to take effect, by which time the patient will probably be quite happy again anyway.

Recently, too, American doctors have discovered that some women who take anti-depressants feel significantly more gloomy just before their period. This seems to be because the amount of anti-depressant in their bloodstream mysteriously halves. No one seems to know quite why this happens; it could be because of fluid retention, or a change in metabolism caused by hormonal fluctuations. Either way, I feel it indicates that chemicals are not always the right solution. As we will see in future chapters, stress reduction, relaxation techniques, acupuncture, massage and dietary changes will help with all the psychological symptoms of PMS.

Let's look at some of the common psychological symptoms of PMS. If you can identify with the feelings expressed here, and if those feelings occur cyclically, then there is every chance you are at the mercy of PMS. Unlike a genuinely depressive personality, a cyclical depressive emerges from her black phase with the sense of having been someone other than herself.

Irritability

'I just feel so scratchy and irritable – it can last for a fortnight sometimes. I barely recognise the person I've become. I snap at everyone, I'm a real bitch at home, and yet a small voice inside me is trying to say, "This isn't really me – help!" ' (Jay, aged twenty-four.)

Irritability, combined with crying fits and even agoraphobia, are all common and difficult symptoms for the PMS sufferer. Agoraphobia, the fear of going out, often results from scratchiness because the sufferer is frightened that she will impose her bad mood on others. She knows that those close to her feel they just can't put a foot right; so, because she fears hurting others, she withdraws rather than risk losing control. The trouble is that even when the sufferer knows her ratty feelings are part of PMS – and even if her partner understands this, the ensuing guilt at what has been said can prove as debilitating as the moodiness itself. A real Jekyll and Hyde scenario!

Anxiety

'I feel awful flutterings in my heart – a sense of impending doom. Everything gets exaggerated. I feel sure my father will have had a heart attack by the time I get home – or that the flat is on fire. Rarely can I pinpoint what I'm actually anxious about – it's just a general sense of something bad about to happen.' (Hetta, aged forty-three.)

Anxiety is a tricky emotion to deal with and live with, because the sufferer can convince herself of the most appalling scenarios without any hard evidence. Hetta's story is typical; real dramas going on inside her head without any explanation to back them up. My own story included a phase when my anxiety was so acute that I would suffer panic attacks. These would occur unbidden, without any warning and often accompanied by physical symptoms. My heart would thump faster, the pulses in my neck seemed as if they would throttle me, I would go hot and cold, have shaking hands, and feel as if I was about to have a heart attack. At times, I couldn't breathe, or felt I couldn't swallow. The instinct was to gulp for air, though one doctor told me that this is the worst thing you can do with panic. Small breaths are better; even more effective, she said, was to wear a paper bag on your head.

I didn't know these were panic attacks, though initial relief was at hand the first time I talked about these symptoms and found I wasn't alone in suffering. That made me feel less weird. I also came to see that the attacks were often caused by suppressing emotions and fears. Once I opened up and talked about what was going on, that 'pressure cooker' effect soon wore off. Likewise, my addiction to coffee wasn't helping those palpitations. Caffeine and other stimulants, as we shall see, can greatly exacerbate many PMS symptoms, both physical and psychological.

Anger

Anne's repeated anger really frightened her. 'I was bloody murder to live with. I'd fly off the handle at any given moment. The children suffered the most because they couldn't understand what was going on – at least my husband Paul had some notion that this was PMS. I remember Ellie was playing up, she wouldn't go to bed, and I could feel this shaking inside me and a sensation like a snake unfurling from the pit of my stomach. Before I could stop myself, I had slapped her really hard on her legs. I feel so ashamed about that. I went through a phase of simply not trusting myself near anyone or anything that was weaker than me.'

If Anne's story sounds familiar to you, you will be pleased to learn that she has curbed her anger. A women's support group helped Anne to learn coping skills for her anger. She learnt not to take on extra stress at this time – be it looking after someone else's children or organising tea parties; she also learnt some invaluable relaxation techniques. Anger is a very difficult symptom to accept; in fact, as an emotion itself, even if justified, anger tends to be frowned upon in our society. For women at home, it often comes to the forefront of symptoms experienced, and Chapter 21, dedicated to mums, may well prove useful.

Depression

'I don't want to see anyone when I'm depressed. Everything feels as if it's in slow motion. I can be fine one day; and the next, I wake up as if swaddled in cotton wool. I become aware of every breath I take, and each one seems like a great effort. I don't want to do anything, I stare off into space. I could shoot those people who say, "Snap out of it!" It's not as if I want this depression. It just seems to settle on me like bad weather. My husband often says that when these depressions end, it's like the sun coming out.'

Julie's story is shared by millions of women. PMS depression often accompanies the physical symptoms of listlessness and lethargy – and, in the same way, a sideline of PMS depression is low self-esteem. The sufferer is convinced she is being a pain in the neck; she can read it in people's expressions, and this gives her even more of an excuse to beat herself up.

It is possible that low oestrogen levels can exacerbate PMS

depression, as can deficiency of B vitamins. What is certain is that 94% of PMS sufferers experience depression – which is a frighteningly high proportion.

Neediness or Paranoia
Unless we are one of those blessed characters, like the old 'ring of confidence' girl in the toothpaste ad, we all, to some extent, experience neediness and paranoia in small doses. Think of those situations when your confidence is at a low ebb – perhaps during a party. You feel uncomfortable in your dress and envy the sleek beauties around you. They ignore you, and you become convinced they are laughing at you. Maybe before setting out for that party, you were desperate for your man to compliment you, even though you felt unlovely . . . These feelings of being unsure of yourself are shared by millions of women and, indeed, men at some point in their lives, and unfortunately PMS can exaggerate them.

Many psychologists are currently banging on about the power of positive thinking and, in this instance, turning your attitude around can really help alleviate neediness and paranoia. It sounds hard to do but repeating 'good' messages to yourself throughout the day can work wonders – for example, 'I am worthwhile and lovely in my own right.' Make a list, too, of your good points – your eyes or hair, your intelligence or capabilities – and remember, we are much harder on ourselves than we need or ought to be.

PMS – SO HAVE I GOT IT?

In summary, if some of these stories made you groan inwardly in recognition, then the chances are you are a PMS sufferer. If you read them and thought, 'How peculiar,' you are probably mercifully free of the syndrome. The only hard and fast rule for identifying these symptoms – which, let's face it, can occur at any time of the month – as PMS symptoms, is that they are present in the premenstrual

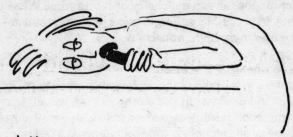

a lethargic sugar craving

phase and that there is a dramatic decrease during the start of a period, for at least a week following the end of that period. Also, that symptoms recur during three successive menstrual cycles. Diagnosis, therefore, depends entirely upon the timing of these symptoms.

You may also have noticed that some of the psychological symptoms I have discussed – for example, anxiety, depression and panic attacks – often occur after a long break without food, but only during the premenstrual phase.

CHAPTER 5

PMS – or Poor Mandy Smith
(the Sorry Stories of Severe Sufferers)

The sheer misery of PMS made life so unbearable for Mandy Smith that she twice contemplated taking her own life. Mandy, teenage bride of Bill Wyman of the Rolling Stones, is one of a number of women who suffer PMS to an extreme degree. Originally, her illness was misdiagnosed as both anorexia and candida. Here is her story, as told to viewers of Thames TV's *The Time, The Place* (13 March 1992), of how PMS affected her life so chronically:

'I wanted to kill myself on two occasions when my weight dropped to five and a half stone. It seemed as if there was no way out. People said it was in my mind. I have got great friends and family who gave me great support and it was only because of them that I didn't kill myself.

'Bill didn't understand. I don't think he wanted to understand it. Even the doctors didn't understand. From hour to hour, my personality would change like Jekyll and Hyde. It would get on anyone's nerves. It got on my nerves.

'It has been the root cause of my problems for seven years. It's misery. It just goes on. Not enough doctors recognise it in this country. It isn't believed. If I can help anybody, even if it's only one person, not to suffer the humiliation I went through, then I would like to. I want to make people understand that PMS is a reality and not something that goes on in the mind.

'The doctors think it was the Pill that triggered PMS because it upset the balance of the hormones. I definitely consider that's what started the weight loss. It wasn't anorexia. The reason I couldn't eat was because of an inflammation of the throat. You have sensitivities rather than allergies, and they cause these inflammations.

'It was very scary. I was changing character from hour to hour. There was a complete lack of understanding from my husband. He didn't have any compassion for me.'

Mandy, now divorced from Bill Wyman, was only diagnosed as suffering from PMS when she visited specialist Dr Katharina Dalton. She is being treated by a Chinese herbal doctor, and is taking oestrogen and progesterone. Part of her treatment involves nibbling every hour so as to keep up her blood sugar level. It is believed that Mandy's extremes of PMS began at puberty when she suffered painful periods.

NICOLA'S STORY

Mandy's case is similar to that of thirty-three-year-old Nicola Owen who, in her book *A Second Chance to Live* (Bantam, £14.99), describes how puberty exacerbated what was to become years of chronic PMS. Nicola made medical and legal history by becoming the first woman successfully to use PMS as a mitigating plea in the courts, when she was discharged from the Old Bailey where she faced arson charges. Dr Dalton also handled Nicola's case. Nicola had turned from a high-achieving, happy child into a moody, suicidal and violent young woman. At the beginning of her problems, her weight soared and she moved from bingeing to starving herself.

Psychiatrists initially thought she was just another anorexic teenager. Nicola then entered a downward spiral, running away to London, frequently blacking out, drinking, attempting suicide, and eventually setting fire to the family home.

Describing her lowest moment, she says: 'I knew I wanted to die. I opened the box of matches and held the flickering light to the curtains until the flames began to dance. Blankly I walked over to my bed and lay down. I turned my head and saw my puppy, Emma, terrified at the door.'

Nicola was arrested and remanded in Holloway prison,

where Dr Dalton linked her behaviour problems to PMS.

Nicola remembers: 'When Dr Dalton started to question me about my periods and the events leading up to them, I was surprised how many things tied into my menstrual cycle.'

Relief for Nicola came in the form of a synthetic progest-erone hormone. Combined with a well-balanced diet of high protein, high carbohydrate, low fat and low salt, plus vitamin and mineral supplements, Nicola is now leading a normal life.

ANNA'S STORY

When Anna Reynolds was eighteen, she killed her mother. She was released from a life sentence in prison by the Court of Appeal after two years, on the grounds that her PMS was severe enough to provide a defence.

Anna had suffered chronic PMS since the age of thirteen. Her symptoms ranged from rashes, black depression, tension and rages to attempted suicide, eating binges, severe breast pain and crippling migraines. Anna had a child by her boy-friend Alan and the child was adopted. She suffered extreme post-natal depression on top of PMS. Her relationship with her mother suffered accordingly. Anna had never seen a pattern to these symptoms, until Dr Dalton helped diagnose her condi-tion.

Anna recalls the day of the attack:

'It was just before my period and I remember spending most of the day in a daze. I was lost in a complete world of my own. I walked across roads without seeing traffic. I always had very heavy periods and always felt dreadful the week before, very unstable, not in touch with reality. I came home from work and immediately my mother started shouting at me. It was an endless stream of abuse: I was a cold heartless slut and I had disgraced the family. I listened, but I never answered back. I wanted to go to bed, but was trembling with something like rage and fear. I went into my room and lay in bed, but she called out for me. In the bedroom on my dressing table lay a hammer. It was there as part of a still-life collection of objects I had been drawing. I grabbed the hammer and killed my mother – that's all I can say. I was so desperate that I completely lost control.'

Dr Dalton tested Anna's blood and came up with conclusive evidence that indicated Anna was suffering from a dangerously low level of progesterone. Her treatment involved injections of pure progesterone for seventeen days each month, until her hormone levels were functioning adequately, and also a three-hourly starch diet.

CRIME OR ILLNESS?

These are tragic stories with relatively happy endings. If sceptics were to argue that such stories are merely illustrative of women exploiting a much publicised and relatively new condition, they might like to consider a few historical facts. As far back as 1845, menstruation-related disorders were accepted by the courts as a defence for a criminal act. That year, there were recorded cases like that of Martha: 'a servant who, without motive, murdered her employer's child, and was acquitted on the grounds of insanity caused by "obstructed menstruation" '.

Yes, there are cases today of women who have exploited PMS to get themselves off punishment for criminal acts, but the true sufferer of chronic PMS who does fall foul of the law never commits her crime in a premeditated way.

PMS is not such a new problem. What is new is that we are more open about it, a fact which has to be welcomed. The old attitude towards menstruation as being something dirty and a 'curse' is thankfully giving way to a more positive, accepting approach. What these stories illustrate is that PMS is a common condition which for some can have life-threatening implications, and should thus be taken seriously.

PROGESTERONE

Mandy, Nicola and Anna were all found to have abnormally low levels of progesterone, a hormone secreted by the corpus luteum of the ovary during the second half of the menstrual cycle. A number of synthetic progestins are available in place of pure progesterone (which can only be given in an injection or suppository). One example, didrogesterone, is relatively expensive and can only be prescribed by a specialist. It is found to be most useful in helping with water retention, irritability and depression. Some women, however, have found that its side-effects include weight gain and a feeling of nausea – which may sound too depressingly like a case of six of one and half a dozen of the other!

If taken as a pill, progesterone will usually be excreted before it has a chance to be absorbed into the bloodstream, and this is why it is usually administered in the form of suppositories or pessaries. The tissue in either the vagina or anus can absorb the hormone into the bloodstream efficiently enough for its effects to be noticed within an hour. There are some reported side-effects; suppositories may increase the chance of haemorrhoids and pessaries may encourage thrush, but these generally occur in women who are susceptible to those conditions anyway. They may also decrease sex drive and cause irregular bleeding.

The Women's Nutritional Advisory Service is rather sceptical about the benefits of progesterone pessaries – but in any case treatments of this nature have been found to be only fully effective when combined with a nutritionally balanced diet, one that involves a regular intake of starch. Given that this is the more natural approach, severe sufferers may like to try a change in eating habits first before resorting to drug therapy (see Chapters 13 and 14).

CHAPTER 6

Calm Down and Help Yourself

There is strong evidence to suggest that many of the popular alternative therapies practised today can alleviate the most common of PMS symptoms. I've included relaxation among them – principally because, in this frenetic world, taking time off does sometimes seem like an 'alternative' practice!

RELAXATION
'When have I got time to relax!'

Relaxation, like exercise, is vital for maintaining a healthy body – and there is growing evidence that both can help to relieve PMS. Both muscle tension, particularly in the neck, back and abdominal region, and the common psychological symptoms of anxiety and irritability can be helped greatly by a regular daily programme of relaxation.

Finding time to relax may sound impossible – especially for young mothers – but even snatching a few moments when your child is asleep (try to make it the same time each day) will do wonders for your well-being. Let's face it, if you want something badly enough, you can usually find time to fit it in. If you're a fan of soap operas, for instance, nothing will stop you from catching up with the latest instalment; well, the same could go for those precious moments spent in quiet, uninterrupted relaxation.

Most of us don't even realise how stressed we are until we

start to relax. I, for one, often go around hunching my shoulders and bunching my hands into fists. It isn't until I consciously relax that I become aware of how stressed I was in the first place. The pace of modern life makes it seem impossible to take time out. Mealtimes, once the focal points of a relaxing hour spent 'en famille', are now usually snatched while undertaking something else. I urge you to try to aim for at least an hour off each day. The benefits will become evident within a very short space of time and, during the premenstrual phase, these benefits will be of vital help to the sufferer.

DISEASE MEANS DIS-EASE

A relaxation technique can be very simple to learn. You won't have to think up a chant, or ponder on a complicated mantra, nor need you adopt some strange contortionist shape on a hard cold floor. Rest is one of the in-built rules of the body, so learning a simple technique is vital as well as helpful.

Did you know, for instance, that the heart, which you might imagine works continuously day and night, actually rests for longer than it works? Every time it beats, there is a rest period for its muscle of approximately 0.5 of a second compared to a work period of 0.3 of a second. Similarly, when the uterus is working to deliver the baby inside, it rests for longer than it works. It needs that rest in order to work efficiently at delivery – and the same goes for the whole body.

In order to cope with the extra stress of your premenstrual phase, relaxation is very much a necessity. But if you do insist that your life is too busy to allow for a conscious amount of relaxation time, then try the following technique, which Laura Mitchell advocates in her marvellous book, *Simple Relaxation* (see the Bibliography). The method is indeed simple; it's easy to learn and can be practised during meetings, while you drive a car – even while you're at the dentist.

COMMON STRESS POSITIONS AND HOW TO RECOGNISE THEM

Head The head comes forward and is often bent right down with the chin tucked in.

Arms Shoulders are hunched up towards the ears and held there. The upper arms hug the chest, and elbows are bent up.

Hands Clenched, or with fingers and thumbs curled into a fist.

Legs If sitting, the tendency is to wind one leg around the other.

Body Held rigid and forward, which often causes back pain.

Breathing Not steady or regular – the accent on the inward breath.

Face Clamped jaws, teeth ground together, lips tightly closed, tongue cleaving to the roof of the mouth.

Eyes Either screwed up or open wide.

Do these symptoms sound familiar? Let parts of your body go limp, and you will be surprised how many apply to you. The body in stress mode adopts these positions more frequently than not. But telling your body simply to 'relax' won't necessarily work, because it's not quite as simple as that. After all, if you don't know how to relax – bar slumping in front of the TV – how can your tense muscles be expected to know how, without definite information?

Far better to give those tensed-up parts of the body specific commands. These commands tell your muscles to do the exact opposite of what they are currently doing.

For example: if your shoulders are hunched up towards your ears, they are in a tense position. The command you should give them is: 'Pull your shoulders towards your feet.' Notice you don't say: 'Relax your shoulders' – that doesn't give any specific information to the muscles. Likewise, if you say: 'Drop your shoulders,' your muscles are likely to jerk back up again in time – a bit like a ball on a piece of elastic. 'Pull your shoulders towards your feet,' is very much a conscious positive command. We then say, 'Stop pulling' and the working muscles relax. Try it – you will soon feel that new 'ease position'.

The sequences you have to memorise for each joint are:

1.   **move** and **feel**
2.   **stop**
3.   **feel**

That way, you are in control of your own body and in charge of teaching it to relax in a positive way, through positive messages which the brain will relay to each stressed part of your body.

CHAPTER 7

Mastering the Relaxation Technique

Work in a room that is comfortably warm – not too cold and not too hot. Your body will lose heat as your muscles learn to relax, and there's little point ending up shaking with cold and getting tense all over again! Aiming for absolute silence is both impractical and unnecessary – we are not in the business of having 'out of body' experiences here, nor of learning some spiritual chant. This technique isn't about mastering some mumbo-jumbo and besides, if you can only relax in total silence, that won't be much use to you in your everyday life.

THE RELAXATION EXERCISE

Lie on the floor, with just one pillow under your head, your legs uncrossed, and your hands either across your tum or along your thighs. (You can work sitting on a chair, too – either with your head resting on a pillow on the table in front of you, and your body leaning forward, or sitting well back in a chair that supports the back of your head and your back. Your forearms and hands must rest on the arms of the chair and not hang over the edge.)

The commands
Shoulders The order is: 'Pull your shoulders towards your feet.' Feel what is happening as you gently do this. Do not pull your shoulders forwards or backwards, and when you can't pull any further down, *stop*. Don't try to hold them down, and

36

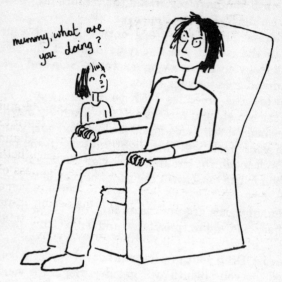

don't be surprised if they bounce back a little – naturally tense people will automatically do this to begin with. Now *feel*. Register this new position of ease. You will probably notice that your neck feels longer, and that your shoulders are much lower than normal.

Elbows The order is: 'Elbows out and open.' Push upper arms slightly away from your sides, but don't lift your arms. Simply slide them away from your body. Gently open the angle at your elbows by moving your forearms (on their support) away from your upper arms. When the position feels comfortable, *stop*. Now *feel* the new position. Concentrate on feeling the 'openness' of your elbows.

Hands The order is: 'Long.' Keep the heel of your hand resting where it is, and stretch fingers and thumbs out as long as possible. Feel the stretch and then *stop*. *Feel* those fingers. They will rest lightly on their support. Feel the pads touching something, the fingers separate from each other. Do not allow them to move until you have registered the texture on which each finger is resting. Take your time over this.

Hips The order is: 'Turn your hips outwards.' Roll your kneecaps out to the side if you are lying down; if you are seated, you will feel your knees swing outwards. *Stop* and *feel*. The same command goes for your knees, too.

Feet and Ankles The order is: 'Push your feet away from your face.' Do this slowly and carefully. If you are lying down, make your feet bend downwards at the ankles and curl your toes. If seated, your heels will rise slightly off the floor, but your toes will still touch the ground. Now *stop*. Stopping will induce relaxation in the muscles in the backs of your legs. *Feel* the result.

Now that your muscles are understanding what it is to be relaxed, lie there for a few moments and enjoy this new sensation!

Face The order is: 'Drag your jaw (or chin) downwards.' Keep your lips closed, or your mouth will get dry. Separate your teeth and leave your tongue loose – not pushed up to the roof of your mouth. When you feel your jaw heavy inside your mouth, *stop*. Feel your lips gently touching and savour this sensation. You may also feel your skin stretching over your cheeks. Feel your tongue loose inside your mouth, touching your lower teeth. If anyone looks in on you, they will probably be surprised at how peaceful you look – for a change!

Eyes The order is: 'Close your eyes.' Do not screw up the muscles around your eyes; think of it as pulling a blind down over a window. Nothing else must be happening to your face. When your eyes are closed, don't allow your lids to flicker or blink. This is something you can learn quite easily with time. *Stop* the movement and *feel* the result. The result should be darkness and peace. Enjoy it and experience the controlled sensation of true relaxation.

Forehead Headaches are common with PMS, often caused by tension and holding your shoulders hunched. What happens is that there is a spill-over of contraction which spreads to the muscles in the forehead, which shorten and tighten on to the skull. It is a bit like having to wear a close-fitting cap.

Relaxing this muscle can be difficult to master, but it is essential to do so if you want a natural approach to curing that headache, rather than resorting to a painkiller.

First, try to concentrate on this area, just above your eyebrows, and think of smoothing it backwards, like a roll-top desk, up into your hair and the back of your neck. (You may feel your hair move while trying this exercise.) Try doing this without raising your eyebrows. It is difficult – a bit like wiggling your ears, I suppose, and this in itself will show you how easily we tense up.

Once you have mastered this relaxation exercise, you will probably become more aware of when and how each part of your body tenses up. This new skill will prove invaluable because you will be able to change your tense position in time, without stopping what you are doing. And don't worry, you don't have to vocalise the commands, so there won't be any funny looks in your direction! Of course, you will only be using the technique partially; for example, a change to the position of your shoulders and one hand while you are working in the office. The main thing is that you are learning to relax effortlessly.

As you can see, these commands really can be done anywhere, without anyone else knowing what you are doing. But probably the best time to do them is before bed. That way, the relaxed state of your body can be kept tension-free for a much longer period of time – and, of course, this new relaxed state will help you to sleep well.

If you do this exercise during the day, have a good stretch of your limbs in various directions before returning to activity. This gives your body a period of time to recover from the drop in blood pressure and pulse.

CHAPTER 8

Exercise

('Exercise? How Dare You Suggest I'm Fat!')

Actually, I'm not – and yes, I agree; the thought of jumping up and down on steps, or thumping your way through an aerobics class, can indeed seem daunting. Daunting really at any time of the month, let alone when your breasts are feeling super-sensitive and your tum is fit to burst out of your leotard. But exercise isn't just about hoping you'll end up like Naomi Campbell; it can also be extremely beneficial for those very symptoms of painful breasts and water retention, and it needn't be so strenuous that you end up feeling completely incompetent after just five minutes.

Gentle exercise is the key to relieving some of the physical symptoms of PMS, especially headaches and lethargy. Similarly, the sense of well-being that exercise brings, not to mention a feeling of achievement that you are doing something positive for your body, can help with the common psychological symptoms of irritability, anxiety, confusion and loss of concentration. Indeed, once you get into an exercise routine that *you* like, you will probably feel irritable if you have to miss out on it for any length of time.

OK, SO HOW LONG HAVE I GOT TO ENDURE THIS?

Aerobic exercising three times a week for at least twenty minutes is the recommended course to take, though if you pick a less strenuous course of exercise, a daily regime of thirty minutes is more preferable. It needn't involve joining an expensive gym; many local councils have swimming pools or gyms that are subsidised – or you can take the even cheaper route and resort to your own two feet for a spate of brisk walking or jogging. But do try to exercise at the same time each day. If you choose early morning, the physical exercise will set you up with enough energy to sustain you throughout the day. Also, the body will get used to this release of tension at a specific point in each day.

My own story is a case in point. I have always found it difficult to wake up at an early hour without the aid of alarm clocks or radios. After joining a gym and forcing myself to exercise at 8 a.m. each morning, I soon found that I woke early naturally – eager, believe it or not, and I barely do, to begin the day with some gentle exercise.

WHAT TYPE OF EXERCISE?

It is essential to find out what type of exercise suits you best. There's no point deciding to become a morning jogger if you loathe feeling out of breath, or hate the thought of people staring at you. Likewise, if you are a very weak swimmer, you could easily get defeated by a course of regular swimming. Find out what you like, and what you are potentially good at. With exercising for PMS relief in particular, it matters less how active you are, how many miles you run or lengths you swim, and more how much you enjoyed the experience. Remember, you are seeking to alleviate those low moods as much as wanting to help eliminate the physical symptoms.

Walking
Americans have now deemed walking a 'new sport' – they have effectively invented it. Of course, I don't need to tell you that walking has been around ever since man first rose to his two feet and put one in front of the other! Joking aside, this is great exercise for people who normally shy away from the thought of exercise in any form. Set aside a good twenty

minutes for your walk and make it purposeful. Aim to get somewhere, via a pleasant route. If you live in a city, a walk to or around the nearest park will be better than pounding the pavements on your way to work. Make sure you are wearing comfortable shoes, and keep up a good pace. Preferably, have your arms unencumbered by handbags or umbrellas, and let them swing in time with your pace. Walking can really aid premenstrual cramps, and also the fresh air will help relieve tension headaches.

Jogging
Don't worry about getting up a good speed. If you pick jogging as your routine exercise, just make sure that you complete the time you have allocated for your jog. Again, comfortable trainers are important but even more essential for sore breasts is a good supportive bra. Jogging does wonders for lethargy and irritability.

Swimming
Swimming has become recognised as one of the best all-round exercises one can take. It works on all the muscles, and given that the water is supporting your body weight, you can work out those muscles without too much of a sense of effort. Don't worry about aiming for Olympic standards – it doesn't matter if you only swim two lengths; the important point is that you enjoy those lengths and that your body is fully exercised in the process. Even more beneficial to specific complaints like water retention and tender breasts is aquaerobics. Many council baths run water exercise classes – they are fun, and a very easy way of working out the whole body in the most effortless manner.

EXERCISE FOR SPECIFIC PROBLEM AREAS

Warm-up routine
Before any exercise, take five minutes out to warm up. This will help eliminate cramps and loosen up the body.

1. Stand with feet slightly apart. Reach one arm up as high as you can, and let your other hand grasp that forearm and literally pull it up towards the ceiling. Hold for a count of twenty and repeat with the other arm.
2. Stand with feet slightly apart. Hold one arm high above your head, and with your other arm travel down the length of your corresponding leg as far as you can reach without straining. Change sides and repeat five to ten times.
3. Sit on the floor with your legs apart. With both arms above your head, breathe and stretch up as far as you can go. Breathe out and reach down towards your right foot. Breathe in and stretch up again. Breathe out and reach for the centre area between your toes. Breathe in, stretch up, then do the same for your left foot. Repeat exercise eight times.

Breast tenderness
A good exercise which helps minimise breast tenderness is as follows.

Stand with feet slightly apart and arms outstretched. Rotate your arms clockwise in a wide circle ten times. Then rotate them anti-clockwise for the same count. Bring your elbows together in the centre, wrists meeting, and hands bunched, and extend arms backwards and forwards to the count of ten.

NB. Some women find it painful to wear bras when their breasts are tender. Indeed, their bra may not fit as well outside the menstrual cycle. A supportive body stocking may help combat this problem – no seams or wires to cut uncomfortably into the flesh.

Cramps
The condition known as dysmenorrhoea spans heavy dragging pains in the abdomen, cramps at the time of bleeding, and lower back pain. The tendency when you experience these sort of symptoms is to tense up and take shallow breaths, both of which are likely to exacerbate the condition. Exercises which

encourage regular deep breathing can really help, as they aid the passage of oxygen-rich blood to the uterus, as well as helping muscles to relax. The following exercises do just that, and can also help your kidneys to work more efficiently, thus aiding the elimination of water retention.

1. Stand straight with your feet together. Place your hands behind your back and lock them together. Bend slowly at the waist, and bring your hands up as high as you can, but don't strain your arms. Hold to a count of five and bring them slowly down while you straighten up.

2. Lie on the floor, feet together. Make sure that the small of your back is firmly pressed against the floor. You can do this by 'cradling' the pelvis upwards. Put your hands either side of your head and lift your head and shoulders off the floor, towards your knees. Don't let your head fall back on the floor. Repeat to a count of twenty, then bring your knees up to your chest and hug them to release the tension. (This exercise strengthens abdominal muscles and helps to relieve lower back pain.)

3. Go down on your elbows and knees, and stretch your upper torso out, lengthening your back so that your head is tucked right under between your arms and your elbows are on the ground in front of you. Hold. This is particularly helpful for cramps.

Shoulders and neck

Tension usually collects at the base of the neck and across the tops of the shoulders. Chapter 7 gives specific relaxation techniques for this area, but exercise too will help to relieve that sensation of tightness. Hunching shoulders in a tense way can also lead to headaches.

Start by lifting both shoulders up and then pulling them strongly down. Repeat this process several times. Then clasp hands loosely behind the lower back and rest them on the buttocks. Keep elbows bent and hands resting on the body. Squeeze your shoulder blades in towards your spine so that your elbows are drawn together, hold and release slowly. Repeat several times.

Remember:

★ If you lead a sedentary life, you are more likely to suffer from disabling symptoms. A more active life will make you feel younger and fitter.

★ You may not feel like exercising in the throes of PMS, so start a regime when you are feeling good – for instance, just after your period has finished. That way you will have become accustomed to it when the symptoms begin again.

★ Wear loose, warm clothing, with support to feet and breasts.

★ Always start with warm-up exercises.

★ Try to exercise each day, and at the same time.

★ Only do those exercises that you actively enjoy – your well-being is as important as the physical benefits that exercise can promote.

★ Don't go overboard at the beginning. You'll end up with stiff muscles and probably feel discouraged.

★ Do not strain your muscles. Work them until you feel the stretch.

★ Give yourself a month or two to establish a regular programme and try not to give up before then. That way, you can gauge just how much the exercise benefits your symptoms.

★ Vary your exercises so that you don't get bored. Perhaps swimming one day, walking the next, and some gentle specific exercises the third day.

CHAPTER 9

Nutritional Supplements

Ultimately you have to judge for yourself whether you think you would benefit from a course in nutritional supplements, since controversy surrounds the link between PMS and supplement deficiency. NAPS (National Association for Premenstrual Syndrome), for example, don't believe that sufferers are particularly low in vitamins or minerals. They point out that the cyclical character of PMS means that the sufferer is entirely well for at least seven, if not fourteen days of the month.

I would say that caution is the keyword here. Vitamins and minerals have proved their worth for a number of symptoms, not just premenstrual, but you need to take the correct dose. Vitamin B6, for example, if taken in excess, can be dangerous and can cause severe nerve damage. Over-the-counter remedies, though helpful, are, I feel, essentially exploitative to women since they are so expensive. PMS, which affects only the female and fertile among us, now offers generous perks for males too, since for druggists there is a fortune to be made from shop-bought 'food' supplements purporting to ease the symptoms of PMS. Evening Primrose Oil, for example, enjoys a market in the UK currently worth £32 million. The problem is that women become so desperate to alleviate their symptoms that if they were offered lumps of coal, they would probably eat them!

My chapters on diet recommend you eat foods that will provide the vitamins and minerals contained in these supplements – and really this should do the trick. Nevertheless, there are advantages to some of the more common supplements available, providing you use your common sense rather than the often high dosages recommended on the package.

EVENING PRIMROSE OIL

Despite its high price, there are plenty of women who will testify to the benefits of Evening Primrose Oil in alleviating PMS – particularly the symptom of breast tenderness – so how does it help?

The evening primrose is actually a humble weed and not a primrose – as we know it – at all. It comes from North America, and gains its name from its blooms which are the colour of real primroses but which open only between six and seven in the evening. More importantly for us, it has seeds which contain an oil high in an essential fatty acid known as gamma linoleic acid (GLA), the same fatty acid that is found in human breast milk.

The importance of GLA lies in the role it plays in helping to maintain the levels of prostaglandins. These are like hormones in the way they work, but unlike hormones they survive for

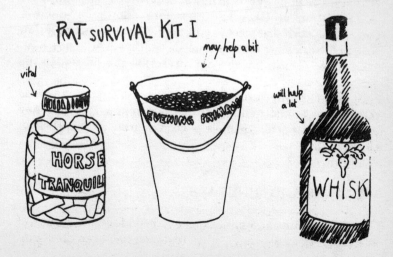

PMT SURVIVAL KIT I

only a few seconds before being destroyed. They are essential for regulating the effects of oestrogen, progesterone and prolactin during the second half of the menstrual cycle – and, interestingly, many women with PMS have a marked deficiency of GLA in their systems.

GLA is produced naturally by the body from linoleic acid, found in foodstuffs like green leafy vegetables, oils, seeds and pulses, and it is important to eat a diet rich in these foods. When the diet is deficient, a supplement like Evening Primrose Oil can certainly offer help – especially for curbing complaints like skin disorders and breast tenderness. Some patients in trials have found it helpful, too, for swollen abdomens, irritability and anxiety.

How much should I take?
Again, it is up to you really. Efamol recommend taking two 500mg capsules twice a day together with a twice-daily tablet of Efavite, which contains vitamin and mineral co-factors. These, they recommend, should be taken for ten days up to the start of your period. Some women, however, have found relief on just two capsules a day, or you could switch to the newer Starflower Oil which has a higher concentration of GLA and therefore allows for a lower dosage. As both are pricey, you may want to start on a low dose and work your way up if needs be. However, if you have a sensitive GP, he or she can prescribe the oil under the name Efamas.

However, having consulted your GP, the first step should certainly be to make sure your diet is rich in foods containing essential fatty acids. Fish is a good source, as I outline in Chapter 13.

VITAMINS AND MINERALS

Specific vitamins and minerals have been found to be useful in PMS but, surprisingly, little research has been done into correct dosage. If you find the following recommendations too complicated, or if the thought of taking hundreds of pills puts you off, look at the dietary suggestions instead. Foods rich in specific vitamins are listed at the end of each section.

Taken to excess, vitamins can be harmful, so if you are pursuing this course, make sure you take the correct dosage. Vitamin B6, as I indicated at the beginning of the chapter, though a well-known aid to PMS, can cause neurological disorders if taken in excess, with side-effects like headaches, dizziness, nausea and restless nights – ironic really, given that these side-effects seem to mirror some of the very symptoms of PMS.

Some experts in the field of nutrition reckon that no vitamin supplements should be taken without medical advice, their argument being that if vitamins did what is claimed for them, then why are doctors still prescribing expensive drugs? Certainly you should be cautious if you are pregnant; on no account take vitamin A or liver products and consult your midwife before taking any supplements. Again, using your common sense pays dividends.

Vitamin B6 – pyridoxine
Vitamin B6 was first used as an aid to PMS back in the early seventies and when taken correctly has been found to help with depression and bloating. In fact, it is known as the 'anti-depression vitamin'. The correct dosage shouldn't exceed 500mg a day, and that should be balanced with magnesium and other B vitamins in order for it to be converted into its active form – for instance, by taking a B complex tablet. Optivite is a multi-vitamin preparation which raises progesterone levels and has a high dosage of vitamin B6. Prescribable by your GP, it has been found to be effective in three out of four cases. Four to six tablets daily, taken ten days before your period, would provide 200–300mg of vitamin B6. Incidentally, vitamin B6 alleviates excess fluid and aids weight loss – another plus as far as PMS is concerned.

FOODS HIGH IN VITAMIN B6
This vitamin is remarkably stable in all cooking methods. Nuts, vegetables, fish, meat, wholemeal bread, porridge and muesli are all high in vitamin B6. A 'Big Mac', on the other hand, contains only 0.02mg of pyridoxine – just 1–2% of the required daily dose. Ever wondered why you feel depressed after filling your face with one? Now you know!

Vitamin B1 – thiamin
Essential for the metabolism of sugar. Higher amounts are needed if your diet is high in sugar, alcohol and refined carbohydrates. If you tend to binge during your PMS phase, then supplement your diet with thiamin. A lack of thiamin leads to anxiety, depression, irritability, aggression and memory loss – and substances like coffee can destroy thiamin. The recommended dose is 1–1.5mg a day.

FOODS HIGH IN VITAMIN B1
These include bread, flour, yeast, pork, potatoes, pulses (peas, lentils and beans) and milk. You can get the correct daily dosage from four slices of wholemeal bread, a bowl of muesli, two rashers of bacon and a large helping of potatoes.

Vitamin B5 – pantothenic acid
The 'anti-stress vitamin'. Deficiency of this vitamin rarely occurs, but if it does, symptoms can include headaches, fatigue, weakness, dizziness, muscular cramps and emotional swings. Poor diet and an excess of alcohol can exacerbate a deficiency. A daily dose of between 5 and 10mg is needed.

FOODS HIGH IN VITAMIN B5
Found in all fresh vegetables, liver, kidney and eggs.

Vitamin C – ascorbic acid
If you smoke, you are likely to be at risk of suffering low levels of this vitamin. The recommended daily intake is about 30mg or the amount contained in an average apple. Increasing your

intake can help your metabolism – in particular assisting the absorption of iron from food – and vitamin C is important for the normal production of sex hormones. If you are deficient in this vitamin, you will probably feel that your energy levels are low, and you may feel depressed, or suffer skin problems.

FOODS HIGH IN VITAMIN C
All citrus fruits and fresh vegetables are high in this vitamin, but cooking can destroy its presence, so eat fresh or raw foods where possible.

Vitamin E
The vitamin found to be helpful for anxiety and depression. Deficiency of vitamin E is rare, but supplements of this vitamin can increase your metabolic rate. Some women have found it helps with breast tenderness too. The recommended dosage is at least 75mg daily throughout the cycle. Vitamin E is unstable and is partially destroyed by any refining or processing of foods.

FOODS HIGH IN VITAMIN E
Dark green, leafy vegetables, wholegrains and seeds and the oils derived from them (make sure the bottle states that the oil contains the vitamin, and don't use for deep frying). Eggs too contain Vitamin E – but only in the yolk.

Calcium and magnesium
In a correct dosage, calcium has been found to be useful for treating cramps, both menstrual and premenstrual. It needs to be combined with magnesium, the body's 'natural tranquilliser', in a dosage of 500mg of calcium to 250mg of magnesium. Some women with PMS have been found to be deficient in magnesium (a mineral found in the body's cells), so they may need to raise this amount. To make matters more complicated, calcium is thought to deplete the body of magnesium.

Magnesium is also necessary in order to make vitamin B6 active, and is involved in metabolism; a deficiency will hinder energy production. It is also vital in the conversion of essential fatty acids into prostaglandins, which are those important regulators in the body needed by every cell and every organ.

If you are lacking in magnesium, and many PMS sufferers have reduced levels, you will probably suffer from a poor appetite, nausea, apathy, tiredness and muscle cramps. It is important for you to consume a diet rich in magnesium, since the chances are that your body is deficient in this mineral during the PMS cycle. Stress in particular uses up large amounts of this mineral, which is also true of zinc and the B vitamins.

FOODS RICH IN MAGNESIUM AND CALCIUM
Good sources of magnesium are nuts, wholegrains and wholefoods, seafood, dried fruits like prunes and apricots, fish and dairy products, vegetables and brown rice. Calcium is found in dairy products like milk and cheese, many nuts, particularly brazil nuts and almonds, sardines, lentils and watercress.

Potassium
Like sodium, potassium is essential for a healthy body – and for helping the cells in the body, particularly nerves and muscles, to function normally. Potassium is best taken through food, since potassium chloride tablets can cause ulceration of the small bowel. Potassium is found principally inside the cells, and sodium outside the cells. The balance between the two is all-important; too much sodium and the body may retain fluid – particularly in the week leading up to menstruation.

FOODS HIGH IN POTASSIUM
Fruit, fruit juices, vegetables (particularly tomatoes), bananas, figs and green leafy vegetables.

Iron
One of the most important trace minerals, particularly for women. It is necessary for healthy blood, and a lack of it can

cause anaemia. It is found in high concentrations in the brain and also in muscles. Deficiency of this mineral is the most common deficiency of all. Symptoms include fatigue, poor quality nails, digestive problems and recurring infections like thrush. If you suffer from heavy periods, then you may be deficient in iron – indeed, an iron deficiency may actually cause heavy periods! A daily dose of 15–18mg is needed and a proper diet can overcome deficiency.

FOODS HIGH IN IRON
Incorporate broccoli, spinach, peas, beans, lentils and nuts into your diet – and if you are a meat eater, liver and beef.

Summary

Vitamins and minerals which directly help PMS:
Vitamin B6 together with a
   B complex supplement   helps depression
Vitamin E   helps tender breasts
Iron   for heavy periods
Calcium/magnesium   prevents mood changes/cramps
Potassium   alleviates fluid retention

CHAPTER 10

Alternative Therapies: from Crystals to Camomile

Old wives' tales – or tried and trusted formulas? You may well be sceptical of anything 'alternative' – and it's not surprising if you are, since the very word does have connotations of weirdo practices. But these therapies, spanning herbal remedies, homeopathy, acupuncture and aromatherapy, have proved excellent in treating specific symptoms of PMS – and if you want to take the natural course rather than resorting to chemicals, it might be worth looking into the benefits of what are, let's face it, ancient cure-alls.

BACH FLOWER REMEDIES

No, it's not a cure which involves listening to organ fugues while sniffing a bunch of roses – the Bach here refers to Dr Edward Bach, an Edwardian bacteriologist and homeopath, who gave up a Harley Street practice in 1930 to devote all his time to research into the healing power of wild flowers. His thirty-eight flower remedies are used today to redress negative states of mind. The doctor was reputed to be so sensitive to the 'energies' of wild flowers that he only had to hold his hand over a flowering plant to sense the properties of that flower. Dr Bach would work himself into a frenzy of negative emotions (he must have had us in mind!) and then wander through fields and hedgerows until he was led to the plant that would restore his serenity and peace of mind. It all sounds like gobbledegook, but let Cynthia speak for Dr Bach:

'I tried everything to alleviate my premenstrual depression. Anti-depressants, which left me sluggish and with a dry mouth; tranquillisers, which made me feel like a stand-in for the Stepford Wives – even therapy. Well, that helped a bit, but the thing was my depression only occurred cyclically, so I couldn't really pinpoint it to a specific event that was happening in my life. A friend recommended I try Dr Bach's remedies. At that stage I was willing to try anything. It all sounded terribly hippy-dippy – even the symptoms listed sounded really weird, like "Wild Oat: helps determine one's intended path in life" – but I was desperate by this stage. I bought some bottles which seemed closest to what my mood changes were, and then put two drops of the remedy in a cup of water which I sipped at intervals. You can also take them as drops directly on to the tongue. I started the treatment ten days before the start of my period, and I can honestly say that it really helped. My husband noticed I was far less scratchy – less likely to fly off the handle – and I didn't have nearly so strong a sensation of bleak despair. They certainly felt more effective than anti-depressants.'

Useful flower remedies for PMS

Symptom	Remedy
Apprehension for no known reason	Aspen
Critical and intolerant of others	Beech
Uncontrolled, irrational thoughts	Cherry Plum
Self-disgust, detestation	Crab Apple
Despondency	Gentian
Pessimism, defeatism	Gorse
Impatience, irritability	Impatiens
Dark cloud, sad for no known reason	Mustard
Fatigued, drained of energy	Olive
Indecision, fluctuating moods	Scleranthus
Utter dejection, bleak outlook	Sweet Chestnut
Apathy	Wild Rose
Resentment, embitterment	Willow

HERBS, OILS ETC.

Today, more and more people are going back to nature to find the answer to health problems, and essential oils and common herbs, as used by the Romans, have made a dramatic comeback. We have discussed the benefits of Evening Primrose Oil in Chapter 9 – but other oils, too, are said to be beneficial for specific PMS complaints.

Starflower Oil

A new product to the natural health market, Starflower Oil is not dissimilar to Evening Primrose Oil. In fact, it contains a richer source of gamma linoleic acid (GLA), the ingredient which is identical to the natural substance produced by the human body to help maintain hormone-like substances known as prostaglandins to keep our bodies on an even keel. Researchers have found that the natural oil from the seeds of the starflower contains 23% pure GLA – more than twice the amount found in the evening primrose. The good news is that you can take fewer, smaller capsules of Starflower Oil and thus save money on this natural course of treatment.

WHAT IS THE STARFLOWER?

The little-known Starflower, also known as borage, is an eye-catching plant with bright purple or blue flowers which attract bees. Its health-giving properties were already known about in Roman times.

STARFLOWER OIL AND PMS

Like Evening Primrose Oil, Starflower Oil works as a GLA supplement. By increasing the level of GLA in the body, it will alter the balance of prostaglandins, which can in turn reduce the symptoms of PMS. Combine this with a diet rich in green leafy vegetables, vegetable oils, seeds and pulses and it will ensure a continuous supply of GLA to the body.

HOW MUCH STARFLOWER OIL SHOULD I TAKE?
Like Evening Primrose Oil, there is no hard and fast rule,
and it really depends on the individual. As Starflower Oil
contains a higher concentration of GLA, its users may need
only one capsule a day. Another source rich in GLA is
Blackcurrant Oil – though it is not as concentrated as in
Starflower or Evening Primrose Oil.

HERB AND OIL TREATMENTS

Fluid retention – or how to blot up the bloat
Juniper Oil (see section on aromatherapy at the end of this
chapter) is said to work on the kidneys and urinary system
(it is also good for cystitis), and **yarrow**, used for colds and
flu, is said to help with fluid retention. **Dandelion**, too, is
said to be a natural diuretic and is very rich in potassium, or
try **raspberry leaf tea**, made from one teaspoon of dried
raspberry leaves steeped in a cup of hot water. **Rosemary
tea**, made fresh, is also good and is said to be effective as an
anti-depressant. **Cucumber, parsley** and **watermelon** are
also mildly diuretic – but simply drinking water may
actually help to reduce bloating.

Chemical diuretics
All these natural diuretic methods are preferable to
chemical diuretics which, though they remove fluid from the
body, can leave the sufferer feeling dehydrated, nauseous,
lethargic and pretty awful generally. Don't be tempted
to take more than the recommended dose of chemical
diuretics even if the albeit temporary weight loss seems
appealing. They can lower blood pressure, sometimes dangerously, and they can deplete the body of potassium. With
too little potassium in your system, you can end up feeling
depressed and weak – symptoms which PMS can induce
anyway, so why bother putting up with double doses of the
blues?

Insomnia

Lavender Oil (see aromatherapy section) is said to work wonders for sleeplessness and also headaches. Put a few drops in your evening bath, or massage into your body at bedtime. **Arnica** is good when you are feeling overtired. **Valerian**, the herbal sleeping tablet, has been proved to be helpful for insomnia – although those in the know stress that it is a very powerful herb and possibly addictive.

Stress/lethargy

Flotation tanks are said to leave lethargy and stress behind. You literally float in a pool of Epsom salts, heated to exact body temperature, and usually in an enclosed dark space, to encourage you to drift off. Health clubs and beauty treatment centres have started to feature flotation tanks – the addition of New Age weirdly wonderful music can be very soothing. Tanks also have a certain radical chic. Margaret Thatcher is said to have survived her sleepless nights by using one, and Ruby Wax has her own private tank – not that they are necessarily desirable role models!

A homeopathic remedy for fatigue is two or three doses of **arnica** (see Chapter 11). And **camomile tea** is a natural relaxant, taken last thing at night. **Passiflora tablets** also help with tension and anxiety.

Nausea

Acupressure (see separate section on acupressure at end of chapter). The ancient Chinese recommendation is to put pressure on the nausea point on the wrist. This involves placing three fingers on a spot from the inner wrist crease moving towards the inner elbow and in line with the middle finger. Another acupressure point can be located by pressing gently inwards on the central midpoint of the stomach, between the breastbone and the navel.

Peppermint tea also helps with nausea, as does an infusion of **ginger**.

Weepiness
Pulsatilla is available from health food shops. (See also Chapter 11.)

Cramps
Mint tea drunk hot can help ease cramps, as does **raspberry leaf tea**. And **sage leaves** are very soothing, taken as a tea, just before bed.

General
Herbalists also recommend **St John's wort** for rest and to aid an increase in energy. **Camomile** or **lime blossom tea** can help with mood swings.

ACUPRESSURE AND ACUPUNCTURE

Chinese medicine has contributed a great deal to female health problems (see Chapter 22). If you have severe PMS symptoms, then acupuncture can be a reliable source of relief, since it appears to stimulate endorphins – the body's natural opiate-like painkillers. It has been found to be beneficial for fluid retention, migraines, backache, painful periods, depression, anxiety and insomnia. Make sure you get help from a registered practitioner – the British Acupuncture Register and Directory keeps a register of practitioners (see Useful Addresses). Generally, however, you will have to pay for treatment from an acupuncturist, unless you are lucky enough to have a doctor who practises the art.

For less severe symptoms, you could always try some self help in the form of acupressure. Also known by its Japanese name, shiatsu, this is finger pressure on specific points of the body – points which are called energy channels. They are the same as acupuncture meridians, but you stimulate them by pressure rather than needles – which will be a relief to those with a fear of needles.

Acupressure works, providing the pressure is right and is

maintained for an appropriate length of time. You also need to learn to breathe properly to get your energy flowing. It might be worth checking at your library to see if there are any local shiatsu classes available or try the Shiatsu Society (see Useful Addresses); alternatively, you can either bribe a friend to help you, or try it yourself. Acupressure can also work by massaging acupuncture points known to help with menstrual problems. Period pains are often relieved by massaging points near the knees, just below the kneecap and in the centre. Rub this point in a circular motion for about ten minutes – yes, it's a long time. If you get fed up or suffer a sore thumb, then enlist the help of that friend.

For depression and anxiety
Pressure points: working along the inner arm, place two fingers two inches above the wrist towards the inner elbow and in between the tendons of the inner arm. Press firmly and hold while breathing slowly.

Period pain
Pressure points: inside the lower leg. Feel for any sensitive points between the calf muscle and the edge of the shin bone. Give these points sustained pressure from the thumb for about five seconds or longer if comfortable. Breathe in a relaxed and easy manner and maintain that pressure until some of the sensitivity disappears.

Headaches and insomnia
Pressure points: the base of the skull. Use your fingertips and work along the area where the muscles meet with the base of the skull. Note any tender points and sustain pressure there until the tenderness disappears. Lean your head back and work your fingers inwards and upwards. Do this along the side of the neck as well, and hold for a few breaths. For frontal headaches, lean the head forwards and press thumbs along the ridge under the eyebrows. Hold, breathe and relax for a few seconds. Working on pressure points along the soles of the feet

and around the inside ankle area can also benefit these symptoms.

REFLEXOLOGY

Foot reflexology is becoming widely recognised as a means of alleviating pain by putting pressure on corresponding points of the foot. Nobody knows quite how it works; some theories suggest that reflexology improves blood circulation and this in turn helps the body get rid of toxins. There are more than 7,000 nerve endings in the foot, and it could be that massaging them helps one to tap into the nervous system and thus release endorphins.

Reflexology has been known to help with PMS symptoms – from backache, insomnia and lethargy to stress-related problems. It is probably better to visit a qualified reflexologist, given the complex make-up of nerve endings in the foot, and The Association of Reflexologists (see Useful Addresses) can put you in touch with qualified practitioners.

Some people have noted that, as with aromatherapy and massage, reflexology can release a lot of emotion – and I'm not talking about getting the giggles from having your feet touched. Be prepared for this and if anything regard it as a good thing – like a release of toxic bad feeling.

AROMATHERAPY AND MASSAGE

Aromatherapy is gaining increasing popularity in Britain today – and not only in the field of alternative medicine. Orthodox medicine is also recognising the benefits to be gained from this natural treatment.

If you have not experienced aromatherapy, maybe now is the time to try it. Treatment involves using concentrated herbal energies in the form of essential oils from plants. These are used in massage, friction, inhalation, compresses and baths. You may find it hard to give yourself a massage, but the very fact that the benefits of aromatherapy can be gained from something as simple as an inhalation or a compress indicates that this is one of the most pleasurable and simple of self-help therapies. Aromatherapy is a holistic treatment, and it can combat a wide range of physical and emotional problems – particularly those that are stress-related.

When you first visit an aromatherapist, he or she will want to know not only about your symptoms, but also about you as a person. You will be asked about your diet, your lifestyle, the stresses and strains of your life – and only then will the practitioner be able to decide which oils will suit you best. Massage with these essential oils forms the basis of treatment, but many aromatherapists will happily give advice on nutrition, exercise and other aspects of your health.

What are 'essential oils'?
No, we're not talking first-pressed extra virgin olive oil – the queen ingredient in foodie chic. Essential oils or essences are not oils in the everyday 'greasy' sense. They are volatile, highly concentrated substances which represent the most

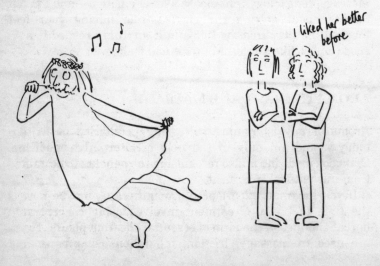

potent form of a plant's aromatic and fragrant materials. They are obtained, usually by distillation, from leaves, flowers, bark, wood and stems. Sometimes huge amounts of raw material are needed to produce just a few drops of an essential oil; for some oils, like lemon for instance, just the zest of the rind is needed.

And no, these oils aren't just pleasant-smelling substances that you can chuck in your bath and be done with – they have specific actions, many of them medicinal, and all to some degree antiseptic, antibiotic and anti-viral. Thus they are able to combat infections, and some have anti-inflammatory properties – lavender, for example, can be used to relieve burns. Many essential oils have a detoxifying quality and can help to clear congestion in the organs and lymphatic system. Still others will act as a tonic – or as a sedative, according to the state of the user.

Essential oils therefore work on all levels. In massage, they work with the skin to heal muscles and organs. At the same time, you are receiving their benefits through smell – and it has been proved that they can activate a deep part of the brain which stores pleasant memories, as well as affecting the nervous system to help reduce anxiety.

How can aromatherapy help PMS?
There are a number of oils which have proved to be really helpful for alleviating specific PMS symptoms. They are as follows:

Symptom	How to use	Oil
Fatigue	bath, massage	geranium, clary, orange, lavender, marjoram, mint, rosemary
Fluid retention	bath, massage	eucalyptus, geranium, juniper, lavender, rosemary, sandalwood

Headache	bath, compress, inhalation, massage	camomile, clary, lavender, rosemary, marjoram, mint
Hot flushes	bath, massage	camomile, lavender
General PMS	bath, compress, massage	clary, camomile, geranium, rosemary
Tender breasts	bath, compress, massage	geranium

As you will see, certain oils are repeated for specific symptoms. Thus, a selection which contains geranium, lavender, camomile and rosemary should suffice for the majority of physical PMS symptoms.

For emotional symptoms of PMS, the appropriate oils can be used in baths, inhalation, massage and as room fragrances. A drop on a hankie can be sniffed in emergencies.

Symptom	*Oil*
Anger	camomile, mint, ylang-ylang
Anxiety	cedarwood, camomile, clary, juniper, tangerine, sandalwood
Apathy	lemon, orange, tangerine, tea tree
Concentration, lack of	cedarwood, eucalyptus
Critical of others	rosewood
Depression	camomile, clary, frankincense, geranium, lavender, orange, tangerine, ylang-ylang
Despondency	juniper
Grumpiness	rosewood
Hopelessness	orange
Hostility	clary, marjoram
Hypersensitivity	mint
Impatience	camomile, lavender, ylang-ylang
Irritability	camomile, cypress, lavender, marjoram, sandalwood, ylang-ylang
Lethargy	clary, cypress, juniper, lemon, orange, rosemary

Mood swings	eucalyptus, geranium, lavender, rosewood
Sadness	marjoram, orange
Sulkiness	clary, rosewood
Touchiness	lemon

QUALITY, NOT QUANTITY

Only the best oils should be purchased, and from a reputable source. The rarest oils can turn out to be quite expensive but because they are so highly concentrated, they will go a long way. As a rule, though, they should not be applied neat. In massage, aromatherapists blend these oils with vegetable oils, called 'carrier oils', and the best of these are virgin cold-pressed oils which contain active vitamins and essential fatty acids but do not have a powerful aroma of their own. The most commonly used carrier oils include walnut, wheatgerm, sweet almond, apricot kernel and hazelnut. You can buy ready-blended oils, but again watch out for quality.

STORING OILS

Essential oils are in effect active substances and so they should be kept in dark bottles and stored in a cool dry place with caps tightly closed to avoid evaporation. They should keep quite well for three months.

SNIFF BEFORE YOU BUY

If it is at all possible, try to sniff the oil before you purchase it. That way you can see whether the oil is agreeable to you and appeals to your nose. The best way is to put a drop on a hankie and inhale it.

HOW TO USE AROMATHERAPY OILS

Massage

Self-massage sounds impossible – 'how will I reach my back?' you ask. Well, you don't have to have a full body massage to reap the benefits – and for PMS symptoms, working on the abdomen and legs will prove just as worthwhile as the whole body. Use light consistent strokes working upwards. When massaging your tum, move your hands in clockwise circles following the flow of the intestines. This can also be really helpful for alleviating premenstrual constipation.

Baths

This is a very pleasant way to experience the relaxing benefits of essential oils and it can also relieve aching tums and tender breasts. Use a ready-mixed blend or add a maximum of eight drops of pure oil to your bath just before you get in. Don't use soaps, foams or other bath oils and keep the windows and doors closed. Relax for ten minutes.

Inhalation/facials

This is an effective way of cleansing your skin, especially if you suffer from premenstrual dryness or spottiness. It can also help sore throats and congested lungs. Use two to three drops of oil to one pint of water. Float the oil on the surface of a bowl of steaming water, and drape a large towel over your head. Breathe in the steam for a few minutes.

For a compress to help alleviate lower back pain, use a pint of very hot water to which six drops of essential oil have been added. Wring out your compress and apply where needed. A cold compress works well for headaches.

You can also sprinkle one or two drops of essential oil on your pillow, if insomnia plagues you during your premenstrual phase. Make sure your skin doesn't come into contact with the neat oil.

Room fragrances

As well as creating a lovely atmosphere, room fragrances can have a good effect on your mood and are therefore particularly helpful with those snappy symptoms of PMS.

You can add a few drops to a bowl of pot-pourri, or to drawer liners and clothes-hangers. Alternatively, sprinkle a couple of drops on to a hot lightbulb. You can also put a few drops on some cotton wool and tuck this behind a warm radiator.

CHAPTER 11

Homeopathy

Somebody may well have suggested you try homeopathy to help relieve your PMS symptoms. One of the advantages of homeopathic remedies is that they can treat both psychological and physical symptoms at the same time – and let's face it, a cure that can help with your irritability as well as your bloated tum has to be worth considering!

But what is homeopathy? Is it all mumbo-jumbo – or is this branch of alternative medicine now getting the sort of recognition it deserves? Given the fact that homeopathy has been around since the time of the ancient Greeks, today's recognition of the practice could hardly be considered to have come a moment too soon!

Basically, homeopathy is the medical practice of treating like with like. That is to say, treating an illness with a substance which, if taken in large quantities by a healthy person, would produce symptoms similar to those of the illness it is used to treat. When minute quantities of that substance are taken by a sick person, it helps the body to throw off the illness – a sort of natural healing process, in effect.

Homeopathy has recently received the royal seal of approval – the Queen, her mother and Prince Charles are all avid fans of this branch of alternative medicine – and though it may not be homeopathy's help in curing PMS which particularly appeals to the royal patients (Princess Diana and the Duchess of York excepted), many PMS sufferers report finding tremendous relief from this branch of medicine.

There are now five homeopathic hospitals in Britain, and some GPs also practise homeopathy. Look in any local chemist and it won't be unusual to find a stock of Nelson's homeopathic remedies on sale; even Boots has recently launched a range of herbal homeopathic medicines. All this is great news if you don't like having to take drugs into your body, or if you hate the dismissive attitude of NHS doctors.

As for the PMS remedies, there are some tried and trusted ones that you might like to consider. Some preparations are known by their abbreviations.

Symptom	*Remedy*
Irritability and moroseness with weeping	Nat. mur.
Over-sensitivity, sadness, weeping	Pulsatilla
Colic and upset stomach	Sepia
Fatigue before the period with pain during the period – particularly a bearing-down pain	Belladonna
Touchiness	Calc. phos.
Tenderness of the breasts	Calc. carb.
Increase in weight	Graphites
Depression	Lycopodium
Quarrelsomeness	Nux. vom.
Exhaustion	Arnica

NB. Calc. carb., Calc. phos., Nat. mur., Pulsatilla and Lycopodium have all proved helpful in relieving headaches, painful breasts, sadness, tearfulness and irritability during menstruation.

WHAT IS LUNA?

'I feel completely loony for at least two weeks before my period,' complains Serena.

One of the newest of homeopathic remedies is currently making great strides in the field of PMS – and, if found to be effective, Luna, or Moonlight, could be used as a single remedy

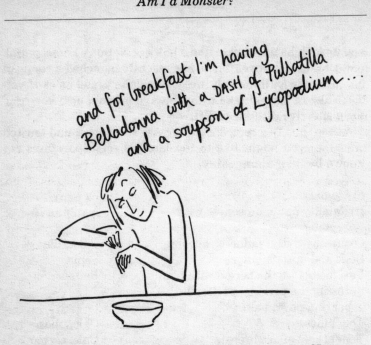

and for breakfast I'm having Belladonna with a DASH of Pulsatilla and a soupçon of Lycopodium...

for a multiplicity of PMS symptoms. The inventors of Luna set up a 'proving' or test-run whereby volunteers were given small doses of the substance and the symptoms produced from taking the 'medicine' were carefully noted.

Luna was found to be helpful for symptoms like irritability, anger, that feeling of vagueness – of being out of touch and unable to cope – in essence, the really nasty, indefinable, 'I hate me' symptoms which plague so many women before their periods, as well as many specific physical symptoms associated with PMS.

A little bit of folklore

Luna does in fact have a lot to do with the moon. The moon, as you probably know, plays a large role in our ancient folklore, not least in our tendency to associate irrational behaviour with the rising of a full moon – hence the term lunatic and its common derivative, loony. Think of the popularity of the werewolf myth. The idea of the werewolf suggests a dual nature in man, whereby he is half ruled by reasoning and moral nature, and half by a kind of animal instinct, usually characterised by unbridled carnivorous passion when aroused. This part of his nature in myth takes precedence when the moon is at its fullest.

So what has this got to do with PMS or, indeed, homeopathy? In homeopathy, there is a strange class of remedies which are often referred to as 'imponderables'. These remedies have been derived not from a physical substance, but from emanations from a radiant source – as 'Sol' is based on emanations from the sun. When an inert substance like milk sugar is exposed to such a source for a period of time, and then this 'charged' milk sugar is potentised, it produces a medicinally potent remedy which can be 'proved' and then prescribed like any other remedy.

An extraordinary story

Luna is just such a remedy. Because of the moon's strong association with the human make-up as well as with the dynamics of nature, a number of homeopaths felt that a remedy made from a substance exposed to the moon's rays might well prove helpful as a medicine for specific psychological complaints. Luna was first prepared in October 1987. Homeopath Melissa Assilem and John Morgan worked with a full harvest moon, using two separate vehicles. One contained ethyl alcohol and the other milk sugar. For a period of six hours, the alcohol was exposed directly to the moon's rays and the milk sugar was also exposed in a crystal bowl and stirred periodically. The two 'vehicles' were later condensed and combined. A 'proving' was conducted using fifteen females and five males, all of whom were healthy before the experiment; each volunteer was given a diary in which to record definite symptoms, whether mental, emotional or physical, over an average fourteen-day period. The results were quite extraordinary. More women than men experienced the following symptoms quite acutely:

confusion/difficulty in concentration
frustration

irritability, snappiness (before period in women)
sadness
emotional sensitivity
lethargy
headaches
gritty, sore eyes
nausea
thirst
tiredness
vivid dreams
pimples erupting on face
increased sensitivity to alcohol

Do these symptoms sound familiar? If you suffer from PMS, you will recognise them as being typical of the sort of 'ills' which plague your well-being before your period.

LUNA'S PROPERTIES

The organisers of Luna's 'proving' came to the conclusion that Luna produces some fairly definable symptoms. In the *mental* functions of concentration, memory and awareness, there was a marked deficiency producing confusion, absent-mindedness and a loss of environmental perspective – i.e. being one step removed from the realm of one's duties and relationships.

Similarly, there was a loss of motivation, a desire to be alone, particularly marked in the female volunteers or 'provers' towards partners and children, and subsequent feelings of irritation, frustration and anger. And, interestingly, one volunteer who normally regarded herself as an impatient person felt more patient and affectionate to her husband and children while taking Luna. Remember the concept of 'curing like with like?' In women the symptoms also seemed to be strongest before and during menses.

In the *physical* realm, female volunteers experienced

headaches, nausea, increased thirst, bloating of the abdomen before menses and tenderness of the breasts. Again, significantly, many 'provers' who were used to suffering PMS symptoms noted a marked improvement during or following the 'proving' – and in all areas: mental, emotional and physical.

In conclusion, Luna could be seen as sharing similar properties to remedies like Sepia, Phosphorus, Natrum muriaticum and Pulsatilla – remedies which I discussed at the beginning of the chapter as being helpful in curing specific symptoms of PMS. If this is so, then Luna will be a tremendous aid for women.

HOMEOPATHY IN MINERAL DEFICIENCIES

One homeopathic practitioner I know regularly treats women for PMS. She believes that any homeopathic remedy for PMS should be accompanied by a celloid mineral therapy. This is a non-drug, natural healing form of treatment based on the belief that many of the symptoms result from mineral deficiencies as opposed to imbalances.

Medical opinion is divided here. As PMS is cyclical, there is no evidence to suggest a mineral deficiency throughout the cycle, beyond the fact that some women do find that celloid mineral therapy helps. The argument *for* deficiencies reasons they occur because of the following:

★ You can be born with deficiencies – or be programmed genetically for deficiencies to develop during life.
★ Both drinking and smoking cause significant losses.
★ Physical and mental stress increases our mineral requirements.
★ Even when absorbed, minerals may not be utilised properly.
★ Poor diet and the way our food is stored and processed can account for deficiencies.

Mineral supplements like Blackmores' Celloids are readily
available from health food stores – but consult a homeopath for
the correct treatment first.

CHAPTER 12

Making a Chart

Yes, it's back to form-filling time – only on this occasion, the 'form filling' is a million miles away from the meddlesome type you need for a mortgage. It is a chart which is actually quite easy to comprehend, *and* it has your own best interests at heart.

NAPS (National Association for Premenstrual Syndrome) recommend keeping a chart of your symptoms for at least three months. By plotting where these symptoms fall you can be doubly sure that they are indeed premenstrual, and it also allows you to see at a glance which symptoms affect you more severely than others, and if a definite pattern is emerging. It is amazing how quickly we forget things like depression once they have passed. The relief of feeling better can actually obliterate the fact that you were gloomy for a full ten days two months ago, and eight days last month – so give the chart a whirl. It will also help you to understand the workings, or misworkings, of your body that much better.

Also, if you have decided to embark on a course of treatment, be it homeopathic, dietary or medical, you will have a record from which you can judge whether that particular treatment is having any effect. After a few months, you will see a pattern beginning to emerge. It is likely that you will experience few symptoms from the time your period arrives until at least ovulation, or the mid-cycle point. If you experience symptoms throughout the whole month, it may be that you are not suffering from PMS at all – in which case, having kept this chart up for three months, you should arrange for a full medical check-up.

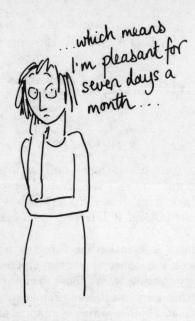

...which means I'm pleasant for seven days a month...

HOW TO FILL IN THE CHART

Fill in the chart at the end of each day, throughout your cycle. Start the chart on the first day of your cycle – i.e. the day that bleeding begins.

For example, a chart for July and August might look like this:

July		*August*
1	d.	d.bl.
2	d.s.h.	d.bl.
3	d.s.h.bl.	D.bl.s.
4	d.s.h.bl.	D.bl.S.h.
5	d.s.h.bl.	D.bl.S.h.
6	D.s.h.bl.	D.bl.S.h.
7	D.s.h.Bl.	p
8	D.S.h.Bl.	p
9	D.S.h.Bl.	p

July		August	
10	p	p	
11	p		
12	p		
13	p		
14			
15			
16			
17			
18			
19			
20			
21			
22			
23			
24			
25		d	
26		d	
27	d	d.h.	
28	d	d.h.	
29	d	d.h.s.	
30	d.bl.	d.h.s.bl.	
31	d.bl.	d.h.s.bl.	

The code I have used is quite simple: d=depression, s=sore breasts, h=headache, bl=bloating, and p=period. If your symptoms vary, you can perhaps use a capital D for severe depression, and so on. Work out your own code, and keep a note of it. You will see I have chosen two letters – bl. – for bloating, because a simple b is not necessarily a good letter to use on its own. You might suffer from backache as well as bloating and be at the mercy of bad mood swings to boot – and if you forget which b refers to which symptoms, it's likely your mood will end up even blacker than before!

It might be handy to keep a note at the bottom of each monthly chart of any other premenstrual symptoms – e.g. panic, chocolate craving, loss of interest in sex, spottiness –

whatever seems to occur cyclically. This chart is also useful for your doctor, for if your symptoms are particularly severe, he or she will be able to see whether a course of progesterone might not be the answer to your problems.

On a separate piece of paper, or preferably in a separate notebook, you might like to keep a diary of what you eat, what stresses you feel, what exercise you have taken, and what emotions you are experiencing. Even noting down anger and resentments – the whys and wherefores – can be cathartic. When you are not premenstrual, go back over your diary and see how you handled the situation. You never know, you may learn something for the next time a bout of craziness hits you . . .

CHAPTER 13

'Food, Glorious Food'

It's time to put away the chocolates, I'm afraid! Come on – you know it makes sense . . .

Actually, we'll deal with those choccy cravings at a later stage, since I know from personal experience that being told something 'makes sense' isn't the way to get me to give up a much-loved vice. I'm a Diet Coke addict – and a former smoker; I used to be able to leave chocolate well alone, but the hell of cutting out smoking saw me reaching for those sugar-packed bars in no time at all! So I know what it's like to have to reform your eating habits – believe me.

Of course, if the following dietary suggestions have no effect on your symptoms after, say, six months, you can return to your bad habits – if you so wish. In truth, what will probably happen is that returning to fatty, sugary substances will make you feel sick, since your body will have been re-educated to receiving healthier foodstuffs. After just one week on this diet, I suffered terrible heartburn when I gave in to my craving for a toasted cheese and ham sandwich and it lasted for forty-eight hours. You have been warned!

Sticking to the right kind of food, for PMS sufferers, is all-important – and that old adage 'you are what you eat' really rings true here. Treatment for PMS is all about making and keeping accurate menstrual charts and aiming for a change in diet which will keep the blood sugar at a higher level. A diet which aims at producing a sustained rise in blood sugar levels throughout the whole month should, by itself, relieve many of the more severe PMS symptoms. It may prove to be all the treatment that is required. Even if you are taking progesterone, the diet must still be followed.

Many PMS sufferers experience hypoglycaemia (low blood sugar) in one form or another. Even if you don't, the guidelines given to hypoglycaemics apply also to general sufferers:

1. It is essential to cut down on fats and sugars.
2. Eat meals on time, and don't skip any.
3. Snacks are essential to provide a level of intake of nutrients.
4. Absolutely no refined foods (sugar or other processed products) and cut down dramatically on caffeine.
5. Take more rest, and learn to control stress.

HOW CAN I POSSIBLY CHANGE THE HABITS OF A LIFETIME?

I know, it's all very well telling you to eat healthily, but those ingrained bad habits are hard to shift, and if you have a family, it can be even harder – especially if your children are picky about certain foods. McDonald's isn't a success story for nothing – kids love junk food, and trying to convince them that a plate of fresh spinach is as delicious as Chicken McNuggets won't always wash. But if you can get them to change their eating habits alongside yours, they will benefit themselves, since the recommendations for PMS sufferers are very healthy lifestyle recommendations indeed. And, of course, it might prove to be the one and only time that your family will benefit from your PMS!

Changing your diet and how you initiate that change is really up to you. You may want to go for the dramatic 'that's it!' approach which has you chucking out any offending refined foods and replacing them with produce fit to grace a health food shop. The way I tried, though longer, seemed a lot less painful – and it has the advantage of being less 'obvious' to the loved ones around you. By gradually introducing certain foods into your daily diet, using them to replace 'bad' foods, you can not only re-educate your palate gently, but also the tastes of your family.

Accept that it is going to be difficult: after all, food isn't just about nourishing the body. Food represents many things – security, comfort, sociability, self-indulgence and reward. If you con yourself that changing your diet is going to be easy and then you find it isn't, you've just created a useful stick with which to beat yourself – something you probably do regularly during your PMS cycle anyway. Don't think: 'I'm giving up' – but 'I'm quitting'. The phrase 'giving up' has such awful implications of deprivation. Even better, concentrate on all the great things you can eat, rather than on the foods you are leaving behind.

You will have to stick with the diet throughout a whole month. Unlike certain supplements – Evening Primrose Oil for example – this treatment has to be adhered to from day one.

Your body may well experience withdrawal symptoms,

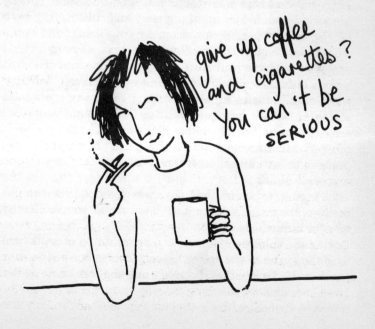

particularly if, like me, you are a caffeine addict. Common withdrawal symptoms from foods range from headaches to lethargy. Take heart, these should disappear after two weeks, by which time your body will have been fully detoxified. Again, taking it slowly, particularly when cutting out caffeine, is probably the least painful way. Why not start today? Cut down your caffeine intake by two cups today, then three tomorrow and so on.

GREAT PMS OFFENDERS

Caffeine Present in coffee, tea, cola drinks and chocolate. Like sugar, it stimulates insulin secretion resulting in a massive drop in blood sugar. Even 'decaffs' contain some caffeine. Sometimes, just giving up caffeine will do the trick – especially if your most extreme symptoms tend to be anxiety, nervous tension, mood swings or irritability. It might be worth cutting down on caffeine before anything else, and substituting herb teas. Peppermint is refreshing as a daytime drink, and camomile as a relaxant in the evening. The range of herbal tea is enormous – find one that suits you best. Redbush is the most tea-like substitute on the market, and you can drink it with or without milk. It tastes a bit like Lapsang Souchong, and comes out looking rather orangey, but you'll soon get used to it. Alternatively, try the new reduced-caffeine PG Tips.

Similarly, try dandelion coffee, if you can't bear the thought of doing without coffee altogether. It tastes a bit wimpish and has a slightly sweet flavour, but for a stronger cup use the roasted root form rather than the instant coffee. You can put this through a coffee filter and in time I swear you will barely notice the difference.

During the summer months, for a refreshing cold drink, you can add a squirt of the new and very delicious cordials (like elderflower) to fizzy mineral water – and that brings us neatly to the second dietary offender.

Alcohol Alcohol contains sugar and, like sugar, has the

effect of causing a drop in blood sugar. In any case, some women experience alcohol intolerance during PMS. Alcohol is a depressant, and its effects can really exacerbate your depression. It is probably well worth avoiding alcohol altogether during the premenstrual phase, but if that sounds too nightmarish, try limiting yourself to one drink a day. It's amazing how much more you appreciate a glass of wine if you sip it slowly rather than gulp it down!

Giving in to alcohol craving can set up a vicious circle for those sufferers who turn to the bottle to help drown their sorrows. Some women experience premenstrual alcohol cravings but the trouble is that those sorrows, under the influence of drink, become exaggerated, not lightened, and given that the recommended weekly intake for women is a mere fourteen units of alcohol (effectively two glasses of wine a day), increasing one's dosage puts the body, as well as the mind, at risk. Interestingly, alcohol can cause hypoglycaemia – and most alcoholics are severely hypoglycaemic – so drinking in your premenstrual phase will only enhance those blood sugar lows.

Sugar Perhaps the greatest offender. Imagine setting a match to a newspaper. The paper burns quickly and ferociously and then dies out – and you need more paper. That is the same effect you get when you fuel the body with refined sugars. You have to replace that quick-burning sugar with a slower fuel – like high-fibre produce (complex carbohydrates). These are found in fruit, potatoes, peas, pulses and milk. Wholegrain bread, pasta and flour should replace refined foods from now on. Introduce fibre slowly into your diet in order to allow your body to adjust, and you should also increase your fluid level – otherwise, strange as it sounds, you run the risk of becoming constipated.

I do appreciate that coming off sugar can be really difficult, especially if you suffer from a sweet tooth, as I do. But there are ways you can help yourself to be weaned off cakes, sweets, chocolate, biscuits and fizzy drinks. Use sugar-free jams and jellies which can be found in health food shops; in the same way, some of the sugar-free nut bars can be used in place of sweets.

Concentrated apple juice can be used as a sweetener in cooking, and if you buy tinned fruit, make sure it's packed in fruit juice rather than syrup. Alternatively, you can try one or two tablets daily of Sugar Factor, a supplement available from Nature's Best which is said to work wonders with sugar cravings.

For food cravings generally, again homeopathy can come to the rescue. Try Ferr. Phos. (Ferrum Phosphoricum) if you get excessive hunger during PMS followed by a complete loss in appetite, or Lycopodium, which is said to be particularly useful when the craving is for sweet foods in particular.

A good test to see whether these dietary changes are working for you is to note whether your sugar craving has disappeared after a couple of months. Like bingeing, you should lose this symptom if you are eating correctly.

Salt This is a controversial one: the general rule seems to be that if bloating is your problem following salt consumption, then cut down. Salt doesn't necessarily cause bloating, however – in fact, there can be as much fluid retention after carbohydrate consumption as after using salt. Some people recommend switching to the low-salt products on the market. Again, caution is necessary since these substitutes are high in potassium and can lead to raised potassium levels, which can be dangerous. Moderation is the answer here.

White flour products Pasta, white bread and other foods made with refined substances should be avoided, though you can have pasta occasionally as a treat – or look out for wholemeal varieties of spaghetti, etc.

SNACKING

I mentioned eating frequently at the beginning of this chapter. This is terribly important. A small snack every two or three hours, as opposed to three large meals and fasting in between, is the order of the day. In women suffering from PMS it has been found that symptoms of panic, migraine and aggression are more likely to occur when there has been a long interval between eating, and also when meals contain insufficient unrefined carbohydrate. This is because adrenalin is at work, pumped into the system to allow the release of glucose from the body's stores. Abnormal adrenalin release is more frequent in women with PMS, and experts like Dr Katharina Dalton have found that adrenalin can be a culprit in blocking progesterone.

You need not make your snacks elaborate or large – a handful of sunflower seeds, a banana, a rice or oat cake, some tofu or half an avocado will do – just enough to top up the blood sugar and keep the internal furnace burning is what you are aiming for. Main meals should have the highest amount of carbohydrate, with a high-fibre element. And if you eat a high-protein snack last thing at night, that will help to fuel you through the night and may indeed eliminate or minimise early morning symptoms.

The best daily plan to follow is:

1. Breakfast: essential! Try to eat within a half-hour of rising and make sure there is a fair amount of carbohydrate from a high-fibre source included in the meal.
2. Mid-morning snack.
3. Midday meal.
4. Mid-afternoon snack.
5. Evening meal.
6. Bedtime snack.

WHAT EXACTLY ARE CARBOHYDRATES?

There are two different types of carbohydrate. First, the refined carbohydrates – those that are low in fibre. These include sugars, foods rich in sugars, foods made from white flours, polished rice, sucrose, sweets and chocolates.

Unrefined carbohydrates are high in fibre. These are found in wholemeal flour and bread, brown rice, good breakfast cereals like porridge and Shredded Wheat (particularly high in fibre), vegetables, fruit and jacket potatoes. When I refer to carbohydrates from now on I am, of course, referring to high-fibre carbohydrates.

And if you are going to take up the exercise suggestions mentioned in Chapter 8, you must ensure that you increase your intake of carbohydrate. Try to eat before exercising – but if this isn't easy, certainly afterwards.

Any healthy body needs a balance between carbohydrates, proteins, fats, vitamins and minerals. Foods high in proteins are meat, fish, cheese, eggs, nuts, milk, pulses and beans.

KNOW YOUR FATS

There are two distinct types of fats. **Polyunsaturated fats** are found in olive oil, soya, sunflower, safflower and corn oil, and margarines made from those oils. Certain fish are high in essential fatty acids, like herring, mackerel, pilchards, sardines, sprats, salmon and whitebait. **Saturated fats** are found in animal fat, butter and milk.

It is polyunsaturated fats that you should aim for, rather than saturated fats. There is a strong belief that a diet high in dairy fats can exacerbate PMS conditions like tender breasts and lethargy, irritability and nervous tension, so keeping your fat level down will help anyway. The fish I mentioned that are high in polyunsaturated fats are allowed, since they will help maintain skin quality and may actually be of value in preventing breast tenderness. It's not without reason that some Evening Primrose capsules contain fish oil: I only discovered this when I got fed up with wresting my capsules from my cat – yes, I kid you not! For a while I believed the cat (a girl to boot) was trying to tell me something – perhaps she had severe PMS? But having read the ingredients, I soon worked out what it was she was after. In fact, if you make sure your diet is rich in these natural essential fatty acids, it will help eliminate the need for expensive supplements like Evening Primrose Oil. I know of one girl who found that Evening Primrose Oil was helping her eczema enormously, but at great cost. Once she started altering her diet to include the right oils, her skin continued to clear, and there were other health benefits.

It is not so difficult to cut down your fat intake. You can, for example, switch from full-cream milk to semi-skimmed, or skimmed if you can stand it, and similarly substitute butter with one of the low-fat spreads. Marks & Spencer has a pretty convincing tasting one called Sunglow, and Olivio will suit those who love the strongish taste of olive oil. Another advantage is that these low-fat spreads don't tend to go annoyingly rock-hard in the fridge, so you can save on your quota of PMS irritability when trying to 'butter' that morning slice of wholemeal toast!

Cut out fried foods if possible – if you have to fry, then do so in an oil high in polyunsaturated fats like soya or sunflower oil. Similarly, choose low-fat yoghurts – bearing in mind that some foods advertised as low in fat are not necessarily that low in fat. The claim should perhaps more accurately be read as 'lower in fat than normal'. Invest in a good non-stick pan and you can 'dry fry' most foods that would otherwise be dunked in hot oil.

There are other 'low-fat' tricks you can employ. Substituting prune purée for fat in certain sweet cooked foods (see Chapter 15) can really help. The purée is both moist and nutritious, and will lower cholesterol levels too. Our recipe for Low-Fat Carrot Cake would, for example, give you only 2.3g of fat per slice, and since it uses wholemeal flour, it is high in fibre too. Yes, the recipe does use brown sugar, but you can, if you prefer, substitute that with a sweetener.

MOOD FOOD

Certain foods play an important role in correcting premenstrual symptoms, especially mood swings and irritability, and I have touched on these in previous chapters. You should aim to incorporate some form of green leafy vegetables or salad leaves into your daily diet. Cook vegetables in the minimum amount of water so as to preserve their vitamin and mineral content.

Uncooked fruit and vegetables are generally more nutritious anyway, since cooking tends to destroy a lot of nutrients. Try to eat at least one raw meal a day – and no, I'm not suggesting something disgusting like a raw liver sandwich or steak tartare, although you can of course eat these if you want – and sushi, the Japanese way with raw fish, is likewise entirely acceptable if that is where your tastes lie. But generally, the sort of raw foods I recommend are crudités, maybe with a low-fat yoghurt dip and a green salad with wholemeal bread for lunch, or a couple of mid-meal snacks of raw fruit.

Eating raw is easier than you think!

CHAPTER 14

'Call It a Diet? Sounds Pretty Fattening to Me!'

Marion was horrified when I suggested that she should switch to a diet high in carbohydrates.

'But it sounds so fattening!' she wailed. 'And I've been desperate to shift that extra half-stone ever since Christmas!'

It reminded me of the woman who goes to her doctor and says: 'Doctor, Doctor! I'm desperate! I'm at my wits' end. I've made my husband's life a misery and the kids are threatening to leave home. I'll give up *anything* if it helps me cure my PMS.'

'Anything? In that case, cut out coffee, alcohol and chocolate.'

'Isn't there anything else I can give up instead?'

Marion's reaction is of course quite understandable. The very word carbohydrate or 'starch' can send the weight-conscious shrieking for cover – I feel much the same. Starch, in particular, has connotations for me of biology O level – those iodine tests we would do on butter-beans and Brazil nuts, vowing under our breaths, as the specimen turned black, to give up doughnuts and other 'starchy foods' for at least a week. Even the word itself sounds horrifically fattening!

The PMS diet needn't be fattening. Cutting out sugars and cutting down on fats is bound to be beneficial to your figure as well as your symptoms, and though you are being asked to increase your intake of carbohydrates, these are from unrefined, high-fibre sources so, if anything, you should be able to lose a little weight, albeit slowly, on this diet. Fat, after all, is the dieter's enemy, unlike potatoes and wholemeal bread. Not only is fat twice as calorific as carbohydrate (nine calories a gram for fat compared to four for carbohydrate), but it is also harder for the body to turn carbohydrate into body fat.

If you do gain weight, it could be that your in-between meal snacks are too large – if so, decrease the quantity and substitute with fruit occasionally. A banana can be filling but not necessarily fattening. Make sure when you start the diet that you are gentle about introducing unrefined carbohydrates into your meals. If you are not used to high-fibre products, you may suffer from bloating, flatulence and wind – hardly symptoms which will help your self-esteem and, if anything, they're likely to cause you embarrassment.

Again, remember to increase your intake of fluids to combat any constipation.

GRAZING AWAY YOUR GRUMPINESS

Interestingly enough, the 'grazing' technique recommended for PMS sufferers – by that, I mean changing over to eating small meals throughout the day instead of the standard two or three large ones – is now being promoted as a healthier dietary approach for any woman. The *Daily Mail* recently talked of grazing as a useful means of burning up fat. Smaller meals taken regularly throughout the day tend to keep blood sugar levels more stable, thus aiding a decrease in feelings of anxiety. Noteworthy, too, is the news that if blood sugar levels get too low, the body produces a spurt of adrenalin to raise the level by releasing stored glycogen from cells – and these empty cells *then fill with water and you get water retention*, so often the bane of the PMS sufferer. So again, grazing can help combat this. The other point to note is that once adrenalin is in the bloodstream, it will stay there for up to seven days and will prevent you from properly utilising the progesterone in your body. That's when PMS symptoms start up. So the rule is once you start grazing, you've got to keep to it rigidly if you want to avoid any return of those symptoms.

And, of course, you must graze on the right foods – those complex carbohydrates rather than choccy bars and bags of chips! And there is a theory, says Wendy Holton, chairwoman of PMS Help, that our great-grandmothers used to eat little and often – and may well have suffered less from PMS than we do.

THE THREE-HOUR STARCH DIET

Dr Katharina Dalton has evolved a three-hour starch diet for PMS sufferers. She conducted a trial, using sufferers who had already been unsuccessfully treated by GPs, alternative therapists, and over-the-counter medicine. Many of these women were used to going for five or more hours without an intake of starch – and a simple alteration in the timing of their diet seemed to bring relief. During the trial period, she found that 23% of sufferers were cured by this diet alone, and 54% found significant improvement of their symptoms. All well and good – so how does it work?

The three-hourly starch regime recommends that you divide your usual food into six small meals, and eat small portions of starch-containing foods (flour, potatoes, oats, rice or rye) every three hours, and always within one hour of rising and retiring. You can eat the rest of your food – the protein, fruit and vegetables – at any time you choose.

Thus, a typical daily intake of food could look like this (tea or coffee should be decaffeinated where possible):

Breakfast
Glass of pure fruit juice, or half a grapefruit
Five tablespoons of high-fibre breakfast cereal (All Bran, Bran Flakes or muesli) or one Shredded Wheat, one Weetabix, or six tablespoons of porridge
Two medium slices of wholemeal bread

Polyunsaturated margarine or low-fat spread
Low or reduced-sugar marmalade
Tea or coffee with low-fat milk

Mid-morning
One digestive biscuit or oatcake
Tea or coffee with low-fat milk

Midday or evening meal
Lean meat or fish
Jacket potato, 6oz
Large helping of vegetables or salad
One piece of fresh fruit or fruit tinned in natural juice

Mid-afternoon
One digestive biscuit or oatcake
Decaffeinated tea or coffee with low-fat milk

Evening or midday meal
Vegetable soup
Two slices of wholemeal bread as a sandwich with:
Meat or fish and salad
One piece of fresh fruit

Bedtime or late evening
Four high-fibre crackers or crispbread
Polyunsaturated margarine
Small helping of lean meat
Milky drink

Remember to drink lots of water too.

This diet would give approximately 1,400 calories mainly derived from a high-fibre source. You can have a daily allowance of one pint skimmed or semi-skimmed milk, necessary to keep up calcium intake.

Obviously, you are going to want variety – and you are probably already asking questions like, 'How the hell am I expected to eat salad without some scrummy dressing?' In the next chapter, I'm going to provide some simple recipes that are low in fat and quite deliciously wicked – carrot cake and brownies, for example!

CHAPTER 15

'While I'm in the Mood'
(or How to Cook Your Way Out of a Crisis)

Here are some delicious healthy recipes you might like to try. The emphasis is on low-fat and high-fibre content. Though it is important to cut down on chocolate and sugar, the good news is that the occasional treat is entirely permissible. These recipes, as you will see, at least have less fat than most shop-bought wicked indulgences. I have also included some good salad dressings. The whole family should find these recipes very tempting to eat, and they are not very complicated to make, so there's no fear that you'll have extra work as well as grumpiness to contend with!

MID-MORNING AND TEA-TIME SNACKS

Low-Fat Carrot Cake

Ingredients
150g (5oz) prune purée (for recipe, see below)
150g (5oz) soft, light brown sugar or equivalent sweetener
175g (6oz) carrots, coarsely grated
3 eggs, size 2, beaten
200g (7oz) self-raising wholemeal flour
1.25ml (¼ level tsp) baking powder
Grated rind of 1 large lemon
Grated rind of 1 large orange
25g (1oz) fresh brown breadcrumbs
Orange slices, grapes and prunes to decorate

Method
1. Pre-heat the oven to 180°C (350°F) Gas Mark 4. Grease and base-line a 900g (2lb) loaf tin.
2. Beat together the prune purée, sugar, carrots, eggs, and 30ml (2 level tbsp) flour. Fold in the rest of the flour with the next four ingredients. Spoon into the tin and level the surface.
3. Bake for about an hour or until just firm to the touch. A skewer inserted into the centre should come out clean. Cool for ten minutes in the tin, then turn out on to a wire rack to cool completely. When cold, decorate with fresh fruit.

Makes one cake (approx. ten slices)

Nutritional analysis
Per slice: 195 Kcals
Fibre 3.7g
Fat 2.3g
10% cals from fat

Prune Purée

Ingredients
225g (8oz) Californian ready-to-eat prunes, stoned

Method
Using a liquidiser, blend the prunes with 90ml (6 tbsp) of water until puréed.

Makes 275g (10oz) 1 cup

Nutritional analysis
Per 275g: 537 Kcals
Fat 1g
Fibre 41g

Prune purée is a good fat substitute for cooking and can lower cholesterol levels as well. Try it in the following recipe for

Low-Fat Fudge Brownies as an occasional treat to satisfy those choccy cravings.

Low-Fat Fudge Brownies

Ingredients
125g (4oz) plain chocolate
150g (5oz) prune purée
3 egg whites, size 2
200g (7oz) soft light brown sugar
5ml (1 level tsp) salt
5ml (1 tsp) vanilla essence
65g (2½oz) plain wholemeal flour
25g (1oz) walnuts, chopped

Method
1. Pre-heat oven to 180°C, (350°F) Gas Mark 4. Grease and base-line a 15cm square cake tin.
2. Break the chocolate into a bowl and place over a saucepan of simmering water. Taking care that no water gets into the chocolate, stir occasionally until the chocolate has melted. Remove from the heat; set aside to cool slightly.

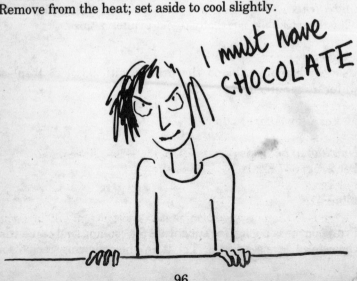

I must have
CHOCOLATE

3. In a separate bowl mix together the next five ingredients. Add the melted chocolate and stir until smooth. Fold in the sieved flour.

4. Spread the mixture into the prepared tin, sprinkle with walnuts and bake for about an hour or until firm to the touch. Leave in the tin to cool completely. Cut into 2½cm (1in) squares.

Makes thirty-six squares.

Nutritional analysis
Per square: 60 Kcals
Fat 1.4g
Fibre 0.8g
21 cals from fat

OTHER DELICIOUS AND NUTRITIOUS TEMPTATIONS SUITABLE FOR LUNCHES OR DINNERS

Herrings with Ginger and Coriander

This recipe is great for those essential fatty acids, and should help with sore breasts and depression. Herrings, steamed in this fashion rather than baked, are quite delicious.

Ingredients for four
8 herring fillets
Freshly ground pepper
4 tsp lemon juice
1 heaped tsp sugar
4 tsp soy sauce
15g (½oz) fresh ginger, peeled and cut into fine strips
Fresh coriander leaves to garnish

Method
1. Season the herrings with pepper and place in one layer in a steamer over boiling water. Cover and steam for two to three minutes.

2. Place the next four ingredients in a small saucepan and simmer gently for three to four minutes. Take off the heat.
3. Arrange the herrings on hot plates and spoon a little sauce over each. Garnish with coriander leaves and serve immediately with lightly cooked vegetables, brown rice or jacket potato.

Baked Brill with Tomato and Herb Topping
A tasty low-fat dish the whole family can enjoy.

Ingredients for four
4 × 150g (5oz) fillets of brill or other fish, skinned
Salt and freshly ground pepper
4 sprigs of flat-leaf parsley to garnish

Topping
2 tbsp freshly chopped mixed herbs: chervil, dill, parsley and basil
1 tbsp freshly chopped chives
60g (2oz) wholemeal breadcrumbs
Freshly ground pepper
255g (9oz) firm tomatoes, skinned, seeded and finely diced

Method
1. Pre-heat oven to 200°C (400°F) Gas Mark 6.
2. Season an ovenproof baking dish and arrange the fish in it in one layer.
3. For the topping: blend the herbs and breadcrumbs in a blender or food processor until combined and uniformly green. Season.
4. Spoon the diced tomato, which must be fairly dry, over the fish and cover with the herb crumb mixture, smoothing the top.
5. Bake the fish for seven or eight minutes, then quickly brown the crust under a hot grill. Garnish with parsley and serve immediately.

Stir-Fry Vegetable Salad

Ingredients for four
1 tbsp olive oil
1 clove of garlic, crushed
1 small piece of ginger, peeled and crushed
½ tsp coriander seed, crushed
1 medium onion, chopped
125g (4oz) baby sweetcorn, trimmed
2 small yellow and 2 small green courgettes, cut into wedges
1 small red and 1 small green pepper, seeded and diced
Freshly ground pepper
50ml (2 floz) rice vinegar, if available
50ml (2 floz) vegetable stock
1 tsp fresh coriander leaves, chopped

Method
1. Heat the oil in a wok or use a non-stick frying pan. Add the garlic, ginger and coriander seed and cook for one minute.
2. Add the onion, then the sweetcorn, then the courgettes. Cook for a further minute before adding the peppers, tossing the mixture continuously. The vegetables should stay crunchy.
3. Season and remove from the heat; add the rice vinegar and the stock, and leave to cool slightly and marinate at the same time. Serve while still warm, garnished with a sprinkle of freshly chopped coriander.

Braised Green Lentils
Lentils are rich in protein, fibre and carbohydrate. Serve as an accompaniment to a piece of plain cooked meat or poultry.

Ingredients for four
255g (9oz) fresh green lentil sprouts
125g (4oz) onions, finely chopped
125g (4oz) potatoes, peeled and diced

40g (1½oz) carrots, scrubbed and diced
40g (1½oz) tomatoes, seeded and diced
275ml (½pt) vegetable stock
1 small clove garlic, unskinned
Seasoning
1 tsp white wine vinegar

Method
1. Wash the lentils sprouts thoroughly.
2. Sauté the other vegetables gently in a non-stick pan, stirring all the time, for about three to four minutes.
3. Add the stock, garlic and well-drained sprouts and bring to the boil.
4. Skim off frothy layer from top, and simmer until the sprouts are just tender, about seven to ten minutes.
5. Remove garlic and season to taste.
6. Finally, add the vinegar and check seasoning again. Serve hot.

Grilled Sardines Stuffed with Fennel and Capers
If you prefer, you can cook small mackerel in this way. Again, a great recipe to combat breast tenderness.

Ingredients for six
12 fresh sardines, scaled and gutted

Stuffing
¼ small bulb of fennel, finely chopped
6 tbsp parsley, chopped
3 tbsp capers, drained and chopped
1 strip lemon peel, finely chopped
Small pinch cayenne pepper
Seasoning

Method
1. Gently sauté the fennel in a non-stick pan until softened a little.

2. Remove from the heat and mix in the parsley, capers and lemon peel. Season to taste.

3. With a teaspoon, gently stuff the sardines with the mixture, then arrange them in a heatproof gratin dish. If there is any stuffing left over, make it into a bed and place the sardines on top. Season.

4. Place the sardines under a hot grill for four to five minutes, depending on their size. Turn over carefully halfway through cooking.

5. Spoon the juices over the sardines when cooked and serve.

LOW-FAT SALAD DRESSINGS

Blue Cheese Dressing

Ingredients
⅓ cup of natural low-fat yoghurt
1 cup of low-fat cottage cheese
1 tsp Worcestershire sauce
1 pinch black pepper
2oz Gorgonzola cheese
Juice of ½ lemon

Method
1. Blend yoghurt and cottage cheese in blender or food processor at high speed until smooth.

2. Add Worcestershire sauce, black pepper and lemon juice.

3. Crumble Gorgonzola and add to dressing, do not grate or blend cheese as it will become bitter.

Makes enough for a salad for six to eight people.

Yoghurt and Herb Dressing

Ingredients
½ cup natural low-fat yoghurt

1 clove garlic, crushed
1 tbsp cider vinegar
1 tsp clear honey
1/2oz fresh parsley, finely chopped
1/2oz fresh mixed herbs and mint, finely chopped
Pinch salt and pepper

Method
1. Place all the ingredients except the herbs in a bowl, add salt and pepper to taste and mix thoroughly with a fork.
2. Add herbs and mix well or blend in blender or food processor for one to two minutes. Chill until required.

Makes one cup.

BREAKFASTS

Summer Porridge
This recipe needs to be prepared the night before.

Ingredients for one
1 cup of porridge oats
1/2 cup low-fat natural yoghurt
1 tbsp sultanas
1/2 tbsp flaked, toasted almonds
1 banana

Method
1. Mix oats and yoghurt to a smooth porridge-like consistency – if too dry, add a little water.
2. Mix in sultanas, and chill overnight.
3. Next morning, sprinkle with nuts and sliced banana, add spoonful of honey if required – delicious!

Winter Fruit Compote
This recipe also needs some preparation the night before.

Ingredients for six
125g (4oz) Californian ready-to-eat prunes, stoned
125g (4oz) dried apricots
125g (4oz) dried figs
125g (4oz) raisins
1 ripe pear, peeled and chopped
1 apple, chopped
1 tsp vanilla essence
1in stick of cinnamon
4 cardamom pods, if available
1 banana, sliced
Zest and juice of 1 orange
62.5g (2oz) flaked, toasted almonds

Method
1. Soak the dried fruit in water overnight.
2. Next morning, drain the fruit and reserve the liquid.
3. Put the soaked fruit and apple and pear into a saucepan with the vanilla essence. Cover with the reserved liquid, add the cinnamon and cardomom pods, bring to the boil and simmer for about fifteen minutes or until the fruit feels soft.
4. Remove the cinnamon and cardamom pods. Turn the mixture into a serving bowl, add the banana, orange juice and zest, stir well and leave to cool.
5. Scatter with the almonds and serve with low-fat yoghurt.

CHAPTER 16

How to Lose Weight *and* Combat PMS

In Chapter 14 I touched on a few tricks to help you avoid cramming in those calories. Now it's time to be more specific because, let's face it, we women are constantly worried about our weight – even if medical experts tell us we are beautifully (and boringly) average in size. I'm not intending to go into the pros and cons of dieting here; in truth, I feel the likes of Twiggy and Kate Moss have a lot to answer for, but there can be few women who would turn a blind eye to piling on the pounds for the sake of maintaining an even temper with their husbands!

But if you want to lose just a few pounds *and* benefit from the PMS diet, this is entirely possible, despite the need for a constant and regular intake of food.

The first rule is to avoid all **fatty foods**.

As I mentioned earlier, once your palate has been re-educated you simply won't like the taste of food heavily drenched in oil. To avoid temptation, hide that frying pan and chip pan, and make a resolution to use the grill instead. Most of the food that you would normally fry will grill just as effectively, with the added bonus that most of the fat will drip out.

What about the **milk** you drink?

Switching to semi-skimmed or even skimmed is not as hard as it sounds. I now can't bear the taste of full-fat milk – and semi-skimmed provides just as much calcium as ordinary milk. Another advantage is that because the fat in it has been reduced, this type of milk won't go off as quickly as the full-fat variety.

Do you like **fizzy drinks**?

If so, try switching to the diet versions – or even better, to plain water. When I gave up alcohol, I decided to go for Diet Coke rather than normal Coke – again, I now cannot bear the taste of 'The Real Thing'!

If you do drink **alcohol**, remember there are lots of hidden calories here. Best to choose a dry white wine, rather than sherry, spirits or beers.

Cheese is delicious, I know – but heavily laden in fat and calories. Opt for cottage cheese, or low-fat Cheddar and hard Stilton. Edam and Gouda are less fattening than most cheeses, and if you like a cheesy taste to your food, use Parmesan as you will need less than with other cheeses to get the same effect.

Vegetables. No restrictions here, but make sure you don't overcook them because then you will be cooking out the vital vitamins. Beans and pulses are great fibre providers, but also quite high in calories, so don't go mad with them. Root vegetables are low in calories and high in fibre; they make a delicious base for casseroles and soups.

Fruit. Though the Department of Health has recently recommended a diet rich in fruit to cut out fat, fruit alone will not provide you with enough unrefined starch to aid relief of your symptoms. By all means use fruit as an addition to breakfast, or as an alternative to pudding, but balance your intake with vegetables, wholemeal bread, pulses, nuts and so forth.

Meat and fish. Fish is much lower than meat in calories and fat content, providing you are not rushing off to the chippie for your fix of cod! Steamed, grilled or boiled is the best way – and in terms of meat, stick to lean meats like chicken and turkey, making sure you remove the skin, which is heavily fat-laden. With lamb or beef, make sure you cut off any excess fat – sadly, it is the expensive cuts that have the least amount of fat.

Each day try to eat:
1 portion of fruit
2 portions of protein: eggs, meat, fish, pulses or cheese

2 portions of fresh vegetables
A portion of starchy food every three hours – including within one hour of waking and one of retiring to bed.

Marks & Spencer have an excellent higher-fibre, reduced-sugar digestive biscuit which could be taken with a cup of herbal tea last thing at night – you could even con yourself into thinking this was some forbidden and delicious treat!

Treats. And as for these, obviously, judge for yourself and exercise caution – but a treat a week won't make you weak!

CHAPTER 17

Men, Madness and Mayhem
(or How to Beat That Bitchiness)

I will be concentrating on your partner's point of view in Chapter 19, giving him space to air his views, but in this chapter, let's think about the two of you, and how you could cope as a 'united front' when PMS theatens your serenity.

The case studies I've included here will illustrate what women want from their partners during these tricky periods, so if your man is willing to read Chapter 19 – and if he does, he will doubtlessly identify with the stories cited – try urging him to read this chapter as well.

Everyone knows that in times of stress, it is usually your nearest and dearest who cops the blame, but knowing that you aren't the only one to take it out on a partner doesn't really help matters much. The feelings of guilt after a long, tearful or bitchy contretemps are almost as hard to handle as the feelings of victimisation suffered by your partner. As with all relationship problems – and this is without doubt a problem to do with relating – in expressing how you feel out of sorts, for example, good communication is of key importance.

Let Shelley speak of her relationship with John, and how the two of them came to an understanding during those hard-to-handle premenstrual days:

'I'm one of those women who seems to get PMS really badly some months and hardly at all the next month. Well, you might expect me to count my blessings, but actually that unpredictability can make matters worse. To begin with, John didn't really think my irritability was down to PMS because I could be sweet as pie another month, with only a bloated belly and sore breasts to cope with, but as our relationship has progressed, we've both come to see that certain outside stress factors tend to guarantee that I'll get PMS that month.

'For instance, we're in the middle of a move right now, and also I'm having to work late at the hairdressing salon most evenings which leaves me feeling very tired. Luckily my best friend there, Lorraine, knows me well enough to know if I'm premenstrual – and she doesn't take offence if I'm short-tempered with her. But then girlfriends are like that, aren't they? They know, because they've been there too. My boss just doesn't understand. He had the nerve to say, "Oh, PMS doesn't exist!" which really made me see red. I felt like chucking in the job there and then.

'Anyway, back to John and me. To begin with – and he is a consistent sort of bloke – he just didn't know how to handle me. It was so obvious that he wanted to be supportive and just didn't know how. He would try to cuddle me, and that would feel fine for about thirty seconds, then I wanted to push him off. "Gerroff!" I'd scream. Of course he didn't know where he stood. It really pisses me off that I can be so foul to him. Once he stormed off back to his flat, and when I rang him and tried to explain that it wasn't him, it was me, he just said, "I wish I knew how I could help." He's so sweet like that.

'Anyway, he seems to have worked out a way, with my help. I told him I would be unpredictable, and that I needed him to be stable when I was like that. It's a lot to ask of him, I know, but he doesn't seem to mind. Now, when I'm premenstrual, he will lie on one sofa, and I'll lie on another – and if I want a cuddle and go over to him, he automatically cuddles me. He seems to be able to sense if I want to be left alone too. I suppose he keeps a low profile really, and that's what works best. And knowing that he doesn't take my bitchiness to heart.'

Not all couples are as lucky as Shelley and John. Julie finds David incredibly insensitive when she's got PMS:

'I know full well I can be a real cow with PMS. Before David moved in – in fact, before we started going together – I could at least confine my moods to a bit of irritability with work colleagues or girlfriends, and the odd tearful self-pitying session on my own – interspersed of course with frequent chocolate binges! But I don't know what it is about close partnerships – they seem to make the symptoms much worse; by that I mean the grumpy, moody, snappy symptoms that leave you feeling and looking, as David often says, as if you've got a face like a smacked bottom.

'Now that David is living with me, I find everything he does a complete irritant when I'm premenstrual. If I come home from work and he's stuck in front of the telly, it can drive me mad. If he doesn't touch me, I want to burst into tears; if he does touch me, I could punch him in the face. Sometimes, he just doesn't seem to realise just how sore my breasts can be at that time; the slightest embrace can have me shrieking in pain, but he just retreats like some hurt dog – or even worse, if we have a row, he threatens to leave.

'I've tried to explain to him that it's all down to PMS, but he doesn't seem that interested. He just says I'm being "unreasonable". I know I am, but for God's sake, I'm not always! I'm normally a very happy sort of person, so you'd think he'd be able to tell this wasn't my normal self. I think in essence that our problem stems from the fact that he takes everything so personally. I really have tried to explain to him, but it hasn't really worked. Nowadays, I just try to clear out of the house if I feel a bad mood coming on, but I know this isn't ideal. I suppose I just want David to understand and be sympathetic – and above all, to not threaten to leave. I feel insecure enough, without that hanging over my head. If he were to step outside of himself and say, "poor you" – even if he didn't feel it – I just know that would help me.'

SARAH'S STORY

'I know I can be an absolute monster when I'm in the full flow of PMS. Unfortunately, my symptoms include migraines – and yes, I get them at other times of the month, but they seem to be so much worse before my period. That has the effect of forcing me to retire to bed; not an easy option when you've got little ones. I have to confess that sometimes I'm almost glad of the migraines. It is as if they give me an excuse not to face up to things: demanding children and a demanding husband. But I know it can be tough for Daniel. Rather than cope with a row, I just retreat. But what I find really difficult about these times is that Daniel starts behaving like a little child himself – and a spoilt child at that. He seems to want all my attention and that's really irritating. Also, strangely, he seems to want sex much more. We have a good sex life, but it is as if he senses I don't want it then, and that makes him want it more.

'The hardest thing for me to take is that Daniel won't accept I'm premenstrual. He thinks I'm punishing him. He either mocks me, and says, "Don't be ridiculous, it's not PMS, you're just using that as an excuse – it doesn't exist," or he goes all hurt on me, and thinks I'm withholding love. I just find that so selfish. What I want is some understanding. I just haven't the capacity to be understanding back – and God knows I've tried. Just a bit of affection would do – a cuddle, and a bit of "there, there"; instead we end up having a row. Now I try to avoid being around him – it's just not worth the aggro.'

Sarah's story is by no means unusual. According to a recent survey conducted by Roche*, nearly eight out of ten men (79%) say their partner goes off sex when suffering from PMS. And 71% of women say all they want is affection and understanding when suffering from the 'monthly blues'. Sadly, less than half the spouses and boyfriends surveyed (45%) realised that the secret to premenstrual harmony lies in a cuddle.

---

* The RSGB study was commissioned by Roche for Starflower Oil. It was compiled from interviews with 900 men and 500 women, based on a representative sample of adults. The base for women questioned was PMS sufferers aged between eighteen and forty. The base for male respondents was men who had heard of PMS, or whose partners were PMS sufferers.

WHAT WORKS BEST

Explaining your mood changes to your boyfriend or spouse at a time when you are not premenstrual is essential if you are going to rub along together the next time your irritability surfaces. The sheer 'distancing' from the mood itself should help you to be more objective and rational in your explanation of your needs – though if you are up against someone who simply doesn't believe in PMS at all, then it will be doubly hard to remain calm and objective during the discussion. Equally, it might be foolhardy to launch into an explanation without any warning that that is what you are going to do. Your hubby may well be happily ensconced in front of *Match of the Day*, and the last thing he will want is for you to interrupt his sports fix with a chat about 'feelings'. At the risk of sounding horrifically sexist, there's no getting away from the fact that, however reconstructed your man might be, explorations of 'feelings' tend to make most men feel uncomfortable. We may bang on about male bonding and mock those denizens of bonding hang-outs – the pub, the gym and the football match – but we women are pretty keen on female bonding too. When women get together, if they click, however short a time they have known each other, sure as eggs are eggs the discussion will soon turn to 'emotional' topics.

PROBLEM-SHARING BETWEEN THE SEXES

Women have always depended on each other emotionally. Look at any situation where they gather: PTAs, the office, the launderette, the shop floor, coffee-break time, and you will find women telling each other about the problems they are having with their husbands, or their kids, their in-laws or their work. Women seem instinctively to know that there is a receptive ear at the ready to listen and commiserate – an ear which will identify with their disappointments, anger and resentment – and, let's face it, their PMS horror stories. Remember

Lorraine's supportive attitude towards Shelley – by no means an unusual case history.

But can the same be said for men with male friends? Somehow I doubt it. Men together do not touch on emotional topics with anything like the same intensity that women do. And isn't it ironic that, despite this, it is also true that most women find it difficult to make their women friends a priority over their men, or to arrange dates with each other without first planning them around the schedules of their men?

Women may depend on each other for certain kinds of personal exchange, yet in our society women's communications are still often devalued and seen as mere chatter, while men's conversations are seen to be of tremendous relevance. Think about your friends, the couples you know and how they interact when they get together, and you will probably find this to be true. The men will raise eyebrows at each other and dismissively label the whispering going on in the kitchen as 'girls' talk'. PMS, periods and anything gynaecological are still sneeringly referred to as 'women's problems'. But we women, on the other hand, will exacerbate the situation by feeling embarrassed if a man hovers around while we are talking to girlfriends. This state of affairs is daft in the extreme, given that the sort of intimacy and understanding you enjoy with a girlfriend is precisely the sort of closeness you need and crave from your mate in order for him to understand you (and more specifically your mood changes), that much more clearly.

BREAKING THE BARRIERS

Sometimes men are jealous of women's friendships – and you can't really blame the poor things! They may well envy the intimacy and ease with which women communicate, and they may wish that they could have a similar closeness with their men friends. Often, too, a man may feel threatened by female friendships and the fact that women together discuss very personal issues with such apparent ease. He may be subconsciously aware that a girlfriend is able to offer things that he feels he can't give to his partner – and he could get to feel resentful about that. Perhaps if you bear these points in mind, together with the knowledge that despite more healthy changes in the way men and women interact, boys do still tend to be brought up not to display emotions, this may help you to see that your problem is about 'getting through' to your man, rather than assuming he just doesn't want to understand. Men and women, let's be honest, are different, and probably always will be.

Your best tactic is to make an 'appointment' to talk with your partner. Yes, I know it sounds a bit weird – but at least this way both of you will come face to face, knowing that discussion of certain topics is going to take place. In fact, this method is helpful for all relationship problems that need airing: setting time aside specifically for discussion helps you to take a more objective, analytical approach rather than the normal, and perfectly understandable, hot-tempered, reactive one.

You will need to explain what is happening to you and how you feel. Also, try reassuring your partner that he is not to blame and that you still love him. You can then suggest ways he might help to relieve the pressure: taking shared responsibility for the children for example, working out a cooking rota, or sharing the shopping – the main thing is to be specific. Hinting, as is our wont, should be avoided – and doubtless the following scenario will ring bells for some of you:

Annabel: 'God, the kids are noisy. I've had them under my feet all day!'
Peter: 'Hmmm, aren't they just.'
Annabel: 'If only I could have some time to myself, I'd feel a lot better.'
Peter: 'I know how you feel. I've had meetings all day – I can barely think straight.'
Annabel: 'They'd probably love to go to the park tomorrow.'
Peter: 'I bet they would. What time are you thinking of taking them?'

Do you see how this indirect form of communication can kick-start a flaming row? No wonder Annabel felt tempted to chuck her tea over Peter, but Peter can't really be fully blamed. If his mind is on other things, he won't necessarily pick up the heavy hint-dropping, hence the importance of making an appointment to discuss specific irritants. This appointment-booking can be done quite naturally, as Lauren found to her relief:

'I could never seem to get Neil to talk to me about my premenstrual mood changes. He was either in a mood himself – blaming me for my faults, or he acted very dismissively or, even worse, he would say, "Don't worry, it's all water under the bridge." I know that sounds hugely sympathetic, but actually it didn't help me at all, because I knew it was only a matter of time before PMS would strike again, and I would end up being irritable, tearful and even violent with him.

'My mood swings were so bad that I actually sought some help from a counsellor, and she told me about how to make a so-called appointment with Neil, so I put it into practice. A week after my period had ended, I said to Neil one morning: "Can we put aside half an hour this evening to talk about a few things? Nothing heavy, but I want to ask for your help with something." That way it sounded bland enough for him not to worry. He agreed, and that evening I broached the subject. I told him that I'd read up on PMS and I knew that it was something that affected me quite profoundly. I told him how acutely aware I was of my mood changes, and how his reactions hadn't really helped me so far. All the time I was talking, I wouldn't let him interrupt. I asked him quite calmly to let me finish talking, and then he could have his say. I explained how I felt that whatever I was trying to suppress usually surfaced when I was premenstrual – work frustrations, money worries, my deep-seated insecurity and so forth. It was pretty vulnerable-making stuff, but to give him his due, Neil listened carefully.

'I also apologised for my anger and violence during PMS and explained how I didn't feel myself at all at those times. I offered a few suggestions as to what would really help me – like being left alone, or him being there for me if I wanted a cuddle – and I agreed that this was a pretty tall order to give, but I just didn't know what else to do. Then it was Neil's turn to talk. He told me how he often thought I used PMS as an excuse for behaving like a spoilt brat, and he felt it a great strain to keep his own temper. When he said that, I really felt wound up, but I had made a deal and I had to hear him out. He offered to read up on the subject, and said he would try his best to be supportive. It was tremendously liberating talking like that – a bit like having a conference!

'Well, the solution has yet to come, but since then, when I get scratchy and he wants to get scratchy back, we look at each other and remember our chat. We call it the "summit meeting" – as in "summit's up with Lauren" – and it can actually make us giggle sometimes, and that defuses the atmosphere. My only worry is that it all seems to be on my terms – but I have told Neil that I'm going to work hard on controlling my anger too, so hopefully that will help matters.'

SHRINK TO GROW

Seeing a psychotherapist or a counsellor, as Lauren did, to help her cope with the depression, anger, irritability and even violent acts that occur premenstrually, might sound like a very drastic measure to take. But psychotherapy has helped countless women to explore the specific emotional issues that upset them at this time. You probably identify with the commonly experienced feeling that your depression is your fault – your irritability is down to your nasty personality or your anger is out of all proportion and probably an early warning signal that you are going off your head – and these feelings are pretty hard to shift when you are in the grip of your premenstrual phase.

A psychotherapist can help you acknowledge and deal with emotions that you would otherwise keep bottled up, and the very best of them can offer practical solutions. By talking to a professional – someone who is not part of your close circle – you may well find that those emotional rock-bottoms are less likely to become overwhelming premenstrually.

Psychotherapy was attacked recently in the press as being a waste of time and money, and accused of offering little advantage over talking to a close friend. If you share similar doubts, bear in mind that it would be a very good friend indeed who would be willing to give up an hour of her time each week just to listen to you. Also, most friends, in a desire to make you feel better, will probably tell you what you want to hear; a psychotherapist would never do that, though he or she will aim to build up your self-love, which is essential for those who suffer from that vicious cycle of anger-guilt-depression. And the sheer fact that you have paid for your session means that you have paid for someone's time and attention – a very liberating feeling indeed! Psychotherapists rarely indulge mere whingers and, conversely, it is often in the protected environment of a therapeutic 'one-to-one' that women first feel free enough to express their anger and needs.

Seeking professional help needn't be scary – far from it – and in the long term, it has to be a healthier option to mind-altering chemicals, thinks Dr Anne Walker, a lecturer in psychology at Dundee University:

'So many women have a concern about being labelled as mad; or they would prefer to say, "I've got PMS" and get anti-depressants from a gynaecologist than say, "I'm depressed" and have to go and see a psychiatrist. Given that many PMS symptoms are so much about behaviour, my own feeling is that they should be going to a psychologist.'

DEALING WITH YOUR ANGER

Anger is one of the hardest of emotions to bear – it's like the top of a volcano, hiding lots of buried feelings beneath. Unfortunately, it tends to burst forth when things get too much to cope with, and so is often inappropriately expressed. We all experience anger, and generally we instinctively know how to control it, but during the premenstrual phase our feelings are often so exaggerated that angry thoughts and outbursts are easily triggered.

There are some useful points you can bear in mind when your emotions are running wild:

Timing

Emotional discussion between couples is often difficult. Because this is so, many people tend to hold back until they feel they could explode before discussing issues. This sort of confrontation turns into a row and eventually it 'all ends in tears', as the saying goes. Some medical 'experts' have described PMS as the time when women tell it like it really is – when they become more honest with themselves. Perhaps if you are prone to shouting at your husband or boyfriend premenstrually, you are really trying to say that you harbour real grievances against him which you successfully suppress at other times. A lot of women do indeed agree that if they are unhappy, the reasons for that unhappiness seem much clearer and more obvious just before a period is due. But if, as I suggested earlier, you make a practice of talking to each other about any irritants in calmer times, then the chances are you will be taking away the 'fuel' which ignites your premenstrual anger.

Telling your partner in the right way

Expressing what you feel is very important, but try to do it in a way that isn't blaming, hysterical, or punishing. The calmer you are, the easier you are to listen to. Obviously, it is pretty difficult to talk calmly in the midst of PMS – hence the importance of setting time aside during your 'normal' phase. What you say will get remembered, and hopefully will help place those inappropriate PMS explosions in their proper context: a case of you not being you!

It can be pretty frightening to find yourself fighting with the one you love best, but ignoring those angry moods is more dangerous than expressing them positively. I say positively, because letting anger dictate to you can have negative effects. It makes you reckless, and can lead you to hit out verbally and even physically – actions you will doubtless live to regret once the anger and the PMS have subsided.

Keeping a diary

In Chapter 12, I talked about the advantages of keeping a diary to help you chart when your symptoms occur. The same practice is useful for listing your angry moments. Note down the incidents that triggered them, and beneath that put down any other feelings you had at the same time. This can include physical feelings like a headache or tiredness. It might read like this:

1	2
depression	sadness
self-dislike	fear
self-protectiveness	guilt
headache	tiredness

This will help you get a better grip on all your feelings, what causes them, and how you can remove the causes of your anger.

Make a list

Make a list of things that irritate you and put you in a bad mood, and underneath each item, write the heading: 'It would be better if . . .', listing what your partner could do to remove the irritation. Under this, put another heading: 'What I could do . . .', listing ways you could reduce the irritation for yourself.

For example:

'When I'm premenstrual, I can't stand watching Ian eat breakfast. The sound of him slurping up cornflakes drives me bananas.

'*It would be better if* he closed his mouth while he ate!
'*What I can do* is have my morning bath while he is eating breakfast and so remove myself from his presence, rather than snap at him.'

VICTORIA'S STORY

'I think anger is all about adrenalin going mad,' says forty-year-old Victoria. 'And you need to discharge that energy – that's why you tend to lash out unnecessarily. Once, I was feeling so angry that, rather than get caught up in a row, I went into the garden and dug a whole vegetable plot! It was incredibly satisfying seeing the good I had done at the end, and it certainly dispersed my anger in a positive way. I think anger can be expressed, but preferably by doing something creative with that pent-up energy. I try to remember this when I feel caught in the grip of anger.'

Remember that super-sensitivity to smells, colours and sounds I discussed in Chapter 3? A surprising number of women feel extra-creative during their premenstrual phase. This can find fruit in a frenzied approach to work, or perhaps

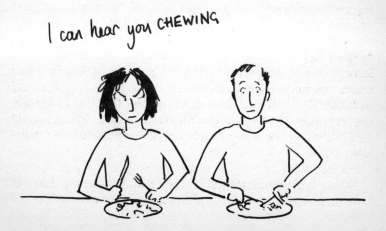

in a desire to draw, cook, write a short story or garden. There is no doubt that in this phase you are usually directed more by what is occurring inside you than outside, and this can stimulate creative expression. If that is the case with you – use it! The result may not necessarily be better than when you are not premenstrual, but it will certainly help to defuse negative emotions. As Victoria says, 'Even clearing out a room, or changing around the furniture can be rewarding and a good way of getting rid of a bad mood.'

CHAPTER 18

How to Find a Therapist

Counsellors and psychotherapists are generally a pretty down-to-earth bunch. They don't all sport beards, unruly hair and round steel specs – nor are they weird eccentrics in white coats. You can even get them on the NHS. But how do you find one that suits you?

Remember that if you do undertake a course of counselling, you are embarking on a new relationship – admittedly different from the sort you have with friends or a lover – but a relationship all the same. In other words, you will, you hope, 'click' with that person. It is of paramount importance that you should be able to trust your counsellor.

Seeking help for emotional problems has thankfully lost its 'therapy schmerapy' taboo – that stigma of the victim, the inadequate person. Most people who go for help are simply fed up with recurring problems in their lives – and, let's face it, we don't hesitate to see a GP for the slightest physical ailment, so why do we shy away from ailments of the mind? You could always ask around your friends first. The chances are that there will be someone in your group who has sought the advice of a professional, and if that friend is 'like-minded' and has found benefit from his or her sessions, then the therapist recommended may well help you as well.

WHO'S WHO IN THE BUSINESS OF SHRINKS

A **counsellor** can help you get over a particular crisis in your life – relationship problems at home, for example. He or she

121

will be skilled in helping you to regain confidence and control of your emotions, and in teaching you to express more clearly how you feel – essential for those PMS blues! Counselling can either be a one-to-one session, or in a group. It is generally a short-term method of help.

A **psychotherapist** generally sees you for much longer than a counsellor would – sometimes for a matter of years rather than months. He or she will aim to help you find the reasons for your behaviour. During therapy you will develop insights into everything behind your actions and emotions, and an understanding of how you can change your actions. Like counsellors, psychotherapists will have undergone therapy themselves, and so will be sympathetic to this unravelling process. This path would be useful if your relationship at home is problematic in the first place, and PMS serves only to emphasise those problems.

HOW TO FIND THE RIGHT PERSON FOR YOU

See your GP and say you want some counselling. Doctors can refer you for NHS treatment – in fact, you can't get NHS

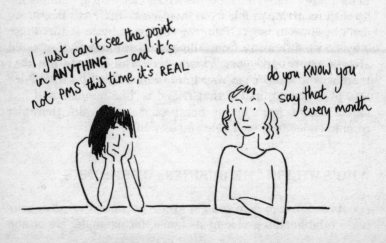

122

treatment without a doctor's referral. If your doctor is not sympathetic, try another one who is.

Try some of the addresses listed on pages 143–145 or contact Relate – your nearest centre will be listed in your local phone book.

WHAT TO DO WHEN YOU HAVE FOUND SOMEONE

You will have an initial assessment of up to an hour, which will give the therapist an idea of your problem. Make sure the therapist understands that your problems are exacerbated during your premenstrual phase (a woman may be more likely to understand than a man).

Feel free to ask about their qualifications: how long have they been practising? Have they had therapy as part of their training? Are they a member of a recognised professional organisation? Ask for a copy of their code of ethics, which should assure confidentiality.

WHAT WILL IT COST ME?

One-to-one therapy Fees vary between £12 and £30 for a one-hour session, but can be higher. Ask if there is a sliding scale of fees, dependent for example on how much you earn.

Group therapy Generally cheaper because more people are involved, but as your problems are connected with PMS, this may not be the best path to follow.

CHAPTER 19

Man Talk

It's the hormones in our bodies,
and the hormones in our lives
that turn women into witches –
and witches into wives.

According to Roche's recent survey, eight out of ten men think women are less competent when suffering from premenstrual syndrome.

★ 56% of men think women are prone to using this widespread condition as an excuse for their bad behaviour.

★ A sheepish 67% of men say that if faced with a monthly period, they would find it very hard to cope physically or emotionally – and, not surprisingly, women agree! 71% of women think men would be absolutely hopeless at coping with periods.

★ 49% of men admit to blaming their partners' moods on PMS, even when they are not suffering.

★ 45% of men say their partners' PMS either puts a strain on their relationship, or leads to arguments.

WHY CAN'T GIRLS BE MORE LIKE BOYS?

Despite the widespread nature of PMS men still remain baffled and confused as to how to help their suffering partners. As Nick says: 'How do I know she's got PMS and it's not just a case of her being moody?'

With some men, the condition is even treated as a joke: 'I

tried to chat up this gorgeous bird last night, but she wasn't having it,' says thirty-three-year-old Jerry. 'I expect she's got PMT or something.'

Or, as sad Robin says in a self-deprecating way: 'I don't know if any of my girlfriends ever suffered from PMS. I just think they all hated me anyway.'

All these comments reveal tremendous ignorance on the part of of male partners – but then, let's be honest: life can hardly be a bed of roses for those men whose wives and girlfriends suffer really extreme symptoms. One minute, you are both chugging along quite happily, and the next, she has turned into a raging, tearful harpy. We may laugh at the very notion of a man having to cope with periods, but imagine being the man who has to live with someone whose mood swings are as varied as Britain's unpredictable weather?

Men's confusion is often understandable and, as in any relationship, it is hard to remain detached, cheerful and bright when the other person is moody, irritable and blaming you. An anonymous letter printed in the journal of NAPS (National Association for Premenstrual Syndrome) illustrates this confusion – *and* the lack of communication that is typical between couples where PMS is an issue:

MONTHLY TERROR OR BAD MOODS?

'As a male living in a household plagued by the dreaded PMT I have slowly become aware of a phenomenon which I will call the "getting to enjoy it" syndrome.

'All the usual horrors of the monthly battles and loathsome hatred for each other are things one can cope with when one knows there is a brief respite to come, but recently the situation has turned very nasty. My girlfriend has always had a slight temper, but now it seems that every little thing can cause a scene.

'As a hopeful writer, it is a struggle to get down to writing as often as I would wish, but the weekend is fraught with danger.

Should I not wish to do what she wishes and want to write instead, there is a scene. Even when I do as she wishes, it is never enough. Maybe she is just insecure or even selfish, I hear you say. That is too simple an answer.

'The loving, caring girl I first met has become so used to being able to blame her tantrums on PMT that now she is relying totally on that one excuse.

'Recently we have spoken of a separation and although neither of us really wants it to come to that, it would seem the only way we can hope to exist as people in our own right. Several pointers prove that this is the only safe course we can pursue.

'Firstly, the monthly fights and rows are rapidly becoming potentially lethal, throwing things and swinging punches – her, not me. Secondly, there is the almost constant fear that one word will start a row. The way I look or sometimes appear is enough to set hostilities ablaze. All these things are blamed on PMT, whatever time of the month it may be.

'Am I the only male who thinks that some women can come to depend on these rows as a way of enforcing their strong need to dominate?

'I am just about at the end of my tether, and can think of no way out of this situation other than the course outlined above. It really is a pity that medical science cannot help couples such as us before things get to this point. Our kids (two of hers and one of mine) often bear the brunt of her moods when I am not home so maybe it's not just me she hates.

'Could it be that as a cynical male I am trying to pass the blame for our situation, or am I simply not trying hard enough to come to terms with her PMT? Some good should come out of this horror or what is there to care for any more?

'Although I believe that leaving is the only answer, I worry that this will not help her to combat the curse of the monthly changes.

'Should I stay and help her fight it or should I run like a scared dog?

'Only those who have suffered what we are going through

will know the feeling of hopelessness, and I pray that some of you can at least understand my turmoil.

'Yours confusedly'

Confusion indeed, but clearly what this couple needs to do is to talk when her moods have abated. It would also be worthwhile doing a PMS chart together, plotting exactly when her symptoms occur. That way, any confusion over whether her moodiness is PMS-related or not would be eliminated – and if it is not due to PMS, she could possibly seek some more appropriate form of professional help.

It is a known fact that illness in one partner can not only put a strain on living together but can cause the break-up of a relationship. When the illness doesn't confine the sufferer to bed and occurs only cyclically, as is the case with PMS, it is sometimes hard for the other person to view the situation as a syndrome which can be treated. Who can blame the poor male who thinks his wife or girlfriend is on a hate campaign or is

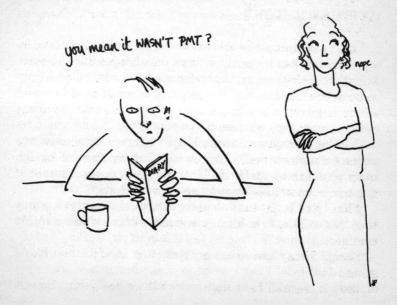

acting like a spoilt brat? No wonder some men avoid coming home if they know they will be met by a fault-finder who sees a box of chocolates as incitement to make her fat, or flowers as a hidden message of a covert affair.

DO MEN GET PMS?

Sounds crazy, I know, but though men do not suffer from PMS proper, if they are living with a sufferer the chances are that they will be affected and involved in the problems that arise, however hard they try to keep themselves on an even keel. There is even one story of a salesman whose sales dropped to zero for one week out of every month. Comparing his sales records with his wife's menstrual record revealed that he was reacting to his wife's attacks of PMS. Once she was correctly treated, his sales record returned to normal.

MATTHEW'S STORY

'I really want things to work out with Sue, for our marriage to be successful, but recently I have found it so hard. I even sought help in therapy – not for me, you understand, but because Sue felt the blame wasn't all down to her, so I was willing to give it a try. Sue is actually very like my mother – highly strung, very emotional – so you would think I would be used to her changes in mood, but I suppose I take after my father, who never really expressed what he was feeling. In many ways I think this is the best sort of behaviour – sure, life is tough, but you just cope and get on with it, don't you?

'What I find really hard to take, though, is that week before Sue's period starts. She can come out with something really hurtful and it just fells me – I feel it almost physically. My face gets hot, I feel a tightness in my chest and I feel as though I'm going to explode. I can't seem to make her happy, and that makes me miserable. At that time of the month, everything I do seems to be wrong. I know Sue feels isolated because I hold everything in rather than let go of my resentments, but how do you unravel a lifetime of stiff upper lip?'

Matthew believes that if Sue's PMS were successfully treated, then all would be fine and dandy between them. Sadly, this hope is all too often a fantasy – putting all the blame of a troubled marriage on PMS doesn't hold water, because even if Sue found relief from her symptoms through diet, supplements or whatever course she was to take, the problems would still remain. In this case, the fact is that Sue needs to vent her emotions and that Matthew doesn't really approve of that sort of expressiveness.

Sometimes, the PMS sufferer finds herself expressing emotions for both herself and her partner – and the explosions, though unpleasant, can be seen as a sort of purge for all involved. When Sue gets angry, it gives Matthew the excuse to get angry back about his own stuff. But if Sue gets in control of her emotions, where is Matthew's excuse or 'prompt' for releasing his emotions? What often happens in this situation is that the couple have to begin to develop new ways of releasing tension – together and individually.

ADVICE TO MEN

Be prepared to discuss the subject in detail with your partner. Read up on the subject and *insist* on her getting some help – not just for her sake, but for the rest of the family.

Try to be patient and caring. If her moodiness and irritability makes you moody and irritable too, then feel free to feel it, but try not to show it. If she gets hysterical, try to be bigger than your fear, and attempt to calm her down rather than admonish her.

Appreciate that she too would love to find relief from this change in her character – she really isn't doing this to attract attention to herself, and the chances are she would like to be welcoming and loving all the time.

Be practical: offer to cook, or take the children off her hands. Tell her you love her, reassure her, cuddle her if that is what she wants. Encourage her to eat something every three hours – small portions of complex carbohydrates will help avoid a drop in blood sugar levels, which can lead to irritability, anxiety and depression as well as several physical symptoms.

Avoid late nights, dinner parties and important functions, which can all add up to extra stress during the premenstrual phase.

Help her recognise she has a problem, and that she can't go round blaming everyone else. Those couples that seem to cope with PMS have a common link in that the man is educated on the subject of PMS, so make sure she knows you understand.

CHAPTER 20

Sex and PMS

Not only can PMS turn normally sweet-tempered, calm females into raging harpies, it can also affect their libidos. A recent survey conducted by the Women's Nutritional Advisory Service revealed that a startlingly high proportion of women who suffer from PMS also get the annoying side-effect of a diminished sexual appetite – and that is hardly a welcome symptom if you are struggling like crazy to keep the home fires burning!

As Geraldine says: 'About a week before my period starts, I can't bear the thought of sex. Besides, my breasts feel very tender – and feeling bloated doesn't help matters either – I just feel too lumpy to be desirable. When I'm like that, all I want to do is hide under the duvet and eat chocolates. But funnily enough, if I time it right, then the actual day before the start of my period, I can feel highly sexed – definitely in the mood for a bit of rumpy-pumpy – and having sex then can actually help to bring my period on.'

Geraldine is not alone in feeling physically and emotionally 'off' sex prior to her period. In a random selection of one hundred PMS sufferers, 60% of women reported that they go through more than a week each month when the very idea of their husbands and boyfriends touching them is quite unthinkable. It is a problem which inevitably causes tension within the relationship. Men, as Sarah's story in Chapter 17 revealed, can feel very rejected by their partner's unresponsiveness. And worrying, too, is that the WNAS survey showed that this problem can get worse with time. Some women reported a lack of libido for three weeks of the month; given they were menstruating for the other week, this doesn't exactly paint a picture of enduring passion. To add to this confusion, many women feel an increase in sensuality during the PMS phase – by that I mean the need to touch and be touched, an increased need for intimacy, be it stroking, holding hands, cuddling or gentle kissing. Not going 'the whole way' can leave an insensitive partner feeling very confused, as he may interpret these overtones of intimacy as sexuality.

One of the most common reactions that partners experience is that the more the woman withdraws from sex, the more he wants it (Sarah's story again) as a reassurance that their relationship is intact.

Again, communication with your partner will help if you are one of those women who suffers a decrease in libido. As a couple develop new ways of talking about PMS and its problems, so any related sexual changes need not be seen as a threat to the relationship, and that couple should be able to be more responsive to each other. And if you are finding success with some of the treatments suggested in this book, your new calmness and freedom from anger and irritability should in turn help you to be more responsive to your partner.

Incidentally, the irritability and relationship problems associated with PMS are not confined to heterosexual relationships. Lesbian women who come forward for help with their PMS often describe exactly the same relationship difficulties with their partners as do heterosexual women – and when their periods synchronise, as often happens with women living in close proximity to each other, then the mix of tension, frustration, resentment and anger can be pretty volatile stuff! What this serves to illustrate is that tensions are not always due to the inevitable differences between the sexes, but tend to be pulled into sharp focus by the sheer fact of two or more people having to rub along together in a confined space. Often, separating yourself from the other person, for even just an hour or so, can really help to ease the atmosphere.

CHAPTER 21

'When I Get PMS, We All Get PMS' — PMS and the Family

It is women who get PMS, but if a woman is part of a family, then the chances are that the whole family will be affected by it too. You may be one of those women who turns her suffering inwards, but if you tend to take out your anger, tearfulness or depression on your family members, what should you do to ease that situation? Once you enter your menstrual phase, and perhaps start to feel more sunny in temperament, can the same be said for your children? They could well be moody and withdrawn for days after your outbursts; they may feel they have to avoid you in case you flare up again. Whatever their reaction, it is bound to make you feel guilty for your earlier actions. Modern parents struggle to play out the role of the perfect provider, and having to come to terms with the fact that they are not perfect is difficult indeed.

And it is significant that PMS has only recently been recognised as a very real condition which can be a potential disrupter of both a woman's well-being and her family life. This is partly due to the fact that more is known about hormones these days, but of equal importance is the changing nature of modern family life. In the past, families were much larger, with grandparents and even aunts all living under one roof. In such an environment, any PMS tension suffered by the mother would have been diffused, as other family members acted as 'buffers' for her black moods. Small wonder that with our nuclear families these moods have taken on much greater significance.

Children, whatever their age, are certainly susceptible to how you are feeling – indeed, from a very early age, they are aware of any mood changes in the family and in those people close to them. Toddlers quickly pick up on an 'atmosphere' of anger or negativity and may soon start to behave aggressively themselves.

So if you are one of those women who gets moody during your premenstrual phase, the importance of a supportive partner who will share the chores of child rearing cannot be overstressed. Having a husband to take the children out for the day will really help reduce your stress. If you have a friend or relative nearby who can 'babysit' or come to your aid, make sure you ask for help, rather than attempt to carry on by biting back your irritation and gritting your teeth.

Alternatively, you can try to offer some explanation to your child which is appropriate to his or her level of understanding. Even a toddler can understand the following statement:

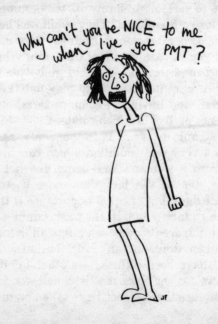

Why can't you be NICE to me when I've got PMT?

'Mummy is not feeling very well today; I'm not angry with you – I just feel angry inside.'

As the child gets older, so your explanation can become more detailed. There is no point in mentioning menstruation if he or she doesn't yet know the facts of life, and actually, even if she or he does, it is perhaps better not to link your explanation of your moods to periods, because otherwise you will be giving the subliminal message that your anger is about having a period, and therefore about being a woman. This will only enhance the stereotypical message that periods are a 'curse' – something nasty and negative. If you have a daughter, this could lead to problems when she herself reaches puberty.

Try instead to see your mood swings as a chance to explain to your children that human beings, and parents especially, are far from being perfect – and that everyone has days when they feel out of sorts. You could encourage them to be more supportive by acting thoughtfully, or by asking if they can help with anything around the house – making a cup of tea for example. This will encourage children to grow into supportive and understanding adults, and on an immediate level will help to take the pressure off you.

If they do ask more specific questions, by all means provide answers, but make sure they are not negatively biased. And invite them to come back and ask more questions once they have had time to think about what you have said.

CHAPTER 22

New Directions

PMS is a persistent condition, and new ideas for alleviating symptoms are constantly being aired. Some of these may well suit you.

SUPPORT GROUPS

'Joining a support group did wonders for me,' says twenty-nine-year-old Juliette. 'Just being able to break that silence with women who understand was marvellous beyond words – knowing I wasn't alone with my condition has really helped too. The trouble with PMS is that you can feel so alone with your condition; until you start to understand the full implications of the syndrome, it is easy to feel that you're going round the bend.'

Many women share Juliette's former sentiment that they are alone in their premenstrual difficulties; many, too, even if they are fully educated in all the facets of PMS, feel ashamed to reveal those difficulties. A PMS support group can provide a safe place in which to share and learn from the experience of fellow sufferers. And before you conjure up images of a circle of women belly-aching (literally) about their miseries, rest assured that these groups offer positive help, even tremendous humour, rather than an excuse for negative navel contemplation!

Society has changed dramatically in recent years and support groups for any problem – tranquilliser addiction, emotional problems, gambling and alcoholism, to name but a few –

have become commonplace. The general accepted belief today is that the value of one sufferer sharing with another is powerful stuff indeed. A PMS support group can also provide a network of women you can call upon when you feel depressed, overwhelmed by anger, and unable to talk to those close to you at home.

HOW DO I FIND A SUPPORT GROUP?

NAPS (National Association for Premenstrual Syndrome) has details of current groups operating throughout Britain; there is even discussion among its members of setting up groups specifically for male partners. You can contact them to see if there is one in your area (see Useful Addresses at the end of this book). Alternatively, if there is not a group already in operation near you, why not think of setting one up yourself?

SETTING UP YOUR OWN HOME GROUP

You could place an advertisement in your local paper or your doctor's surgery, health club or library, expressing your desire to start a group. NAPS will give advice on how the group should be run, but the onus needn't rest entirely on you – starting up a support group isn't about becoming big boss or put-upon tea-lady. You can rotate where the meetings take place; one week your home, the next, another member's home, for example. If you want to separate the group from the home environment, church halls are often very cheap to hire. The vicar or church secretary will advise you, and the expense can be shared by passing round a pot at the end of the meeting. Any leftovers can pay for tea, herbal of course, and healthy snacks.

Once your group is established, be sure to set up a network of telephone support, so that each of you can call up members during times of crisis.

Structure the group so that everyone gets a chance to speak – if the group is large, you will need to encourage members to confine their speaking to five or ten minutes – and you might like to invite a speaker to talk about her experience as a kick-off to the meeting. Encourage that speaker to talk about the positive help she has found, rather than dwelling on the negative. Try to discourage members from interrupting, taking charge, or telling others to 'snap out of it' – not that this is likely with genuine sufferers, but you have probably all come across the 'committee queen', the sort of woman who loves nothing more than trying to control the lives of others. If you haven't, just listen to Mrs Snell in *The Archers*, and that should give you some idea of how important it is to see these groups as a place where equality rules! That said, by all means have a group structure, which can be rotated over a period of time. Elect a secretary, a treasurer, a tea-lady and a greeter, for example.

You may want to learn about alternative therapies as a group. Perhaps one of you has experience as a masseuse or an aromatherapist. Your meetings could then take on a practical and beneficial aspect, with half the time devoted to instruction and discussion of the benefits of, say, massage, the other to group sharing.

OTHER SUGGESTIONS

Chinese Medicine

'PMS? I've never had it!' Lei, a twenty-six-year-old Chinese beauty, looked justifiably smug. 'I can remember my mother forcing foul-tasting herbal tea down my throat from the age of about eleven onwards. I suppose that is when my periods started. I never really knew what went in that tea, but she assured me I wouldn't have trouble with my menstruation if I drank it. I suppose I thought it was the Chinese equivalent of your mother forcing you to eat your crusts to make your hair curl, only in this case it obviously really helped me. My sisters were given it too, and I know they've never had PMS. The more I read about the condition, the more I thank my mother for those horrible teas!'

Traditional Chinese medicine if fast gaining the recognition it deserves, and if Lei's story is anything to go by, this branch of alternative health care can prove to be of immense help to PMS sufferers. Her mother wisely nipped any potential problem in the bud, so to speak, but as Ruth Delman of London's Chi Clinic told me: 'Traditional Chinese medicine can certainly help with women's problems because it's all about treating the whole body. We specialise in skin complaints at this clinic – well, one of the symptoms of PMS is that the skin often gets worse just before a period. Even the menopausal woman's hot flushes can be manifested as a skin problem. We are beginning to specialise in women's problems in particular, and there are a number of herbs that will be useful for the PMS woman. Dang Gui is one – better known in the West as angelica root – which would be taken alongside other herbs, like Bai Shaeo or peony root, Yu Jin (turmeric tuber), Wu Wei Zi (schisandra fruit) and Xiang Fu (nut grass rhizome) in a concoction – usually a tea. Whereas Western herbalists tend to use one, two or three specific herbs for one complaint, the Chinese give the patient a general tonic, and then add specific herbs, specially selected for that individual and according to the symptoms most prevalent. This could be for the stomach, or skin or the gynaecological system.'

Obviously, given the tailor-made nature of Chinese medicine, treatment for PMS would need to be prescribed by a Chinese doctor, and my list of useful addresses at the end of this book will be of help.

The WNAS

'We're not educated about our bodies,' says Maryon Stewart of the Women's Nutritional Advisory Service. 'We don't know what they need.' Diet is of key importance in treating PMS, thinks the WNAS – a service set up in 1984 to provide a holistic programme for PMS sufferers. Since its early days, the response from sufferers has been enormous, and Maryon Stewart sometimes receives up to 600 letters a day from women who are desperate for help. As well as running clinics in London, Hove and Lewes (see Useful Addresses) the WNAS now also has a postal programme (£86, or budget: £48 at the time of writing) where patients fill out a detailed lifestyle questionnaire which provides the basis for individual treatment. Each woman is given a diet very similar to the one recommended in this book, together with supplements like Optivite (containing vitamins B6, B complex, magnesium, etc.) and recommendations for exercise and relaxation; she is then monitored closely by phone or mail over four months. The success rate is high – 95.6% of patients report that their symptoms have either disappeared or improved significantly after three months – so clearly the holistic self-help approach looks like being the way forward.

CHAPTER 23

Conclusion: the Non-Believers
(or PMT, 'Pompous Male Twits')

In spring 1993, the *Sun* newspaper came to the defence of the premenstrual woman. Yes, I know it sounds hard to believe, but the *Sun*'s talent as top tabloid for hitting Achilles' heels was in force with 'Pompous Male Twit', a headline accompanying a leader article which attacked a dissenting psychologist. That psychologist was one of a band of PMS non-believers who consider PMS to be all in the mind. At a conference that spring for the British Psychological Society, top psychologists claimed that women use PMS as an excuse for bad behaviour. These 'experts' said it had become a universal women's excuse, blamed for anything from 'depression to car crashes'. One doctor even went so far as to say that PMS had more to do with being neurotic, and that though a small percentage of women suffered a genuine hormonal imbalance, PMS was usually considered to be psychological.

This sort of unhelpful attitude is enough to make millions of female sufferers feel even bluer than they normally do premenstrually, and the *Sun* has to be congratulated for pointing out the significant fact that these are the opinions in general of men, not women. But PMS *is* a genuine complaint and, as this book has shown, there are plenty of genuine ways in which the condition can be cured.

An effective treatment for PMS has been a long time coming, mainly due to doctors' ignorance or reluctance to diagnose it as a genuine condition. There is even a story of a woman who consulted her doctor for PMS and he advised her to have a baby. When she asked what she should do once she had got the baby, he shouted at her, 'You women are all the same. We give advice and you don't take it!'

Many doctors continue to see PMS as a psychiatric disorder, prescribing tranquillisers and hormones to treat it – and in the past, some doctors would resort to extremes like hysterectomies, ECT and even lobotomies. But though theories come and go and controversies may rage, what of the future? Is there one tried and trusted remedy that will banish those monthly blues for good?

Dr Alan Stewart of the Women's Nutritional Advisory Service reckons there are two methods that will prove the most valuable for curing PMS – and, even here, the one that in his opinion wins hands down is self help.

'One is to change the diet of the sufferer, and this can sometimes mean a really big dramatic change. But with the psychological symptoms of PMS, or when you've got a really chronic sufferer, sometimes doctors are quick to prescribe chemicals which will "switch off" the hormones. Huge amounts of oestrogen, for example, will literally switch off the ovaries, and you can then guarantee the sufferer won't have PMS. But what she will have is perhaps an artificial menopause, or an addictive cycle whereby the sufferer can't do without that prop. In my opinion, the only way forward is to turn to self help measures.'

And that, in a nutshell, is my opinion too!

Useful Addresses

CHINESE MEDICINE

Register of Chinese Medicine,
  19 Trinity Road,
  London N2 8JJ
  (081 883 8431)
  Send SAE and £2.50 for directory of practitioners.

The Chinese Medical Centre,
  Manvers Chambers,
  Manvers Street,
  Bath BA1 1TE
  (0225 483393)

The Chi Skin Clinics,
  Riverbank House,
  Putney Bridge Approach North,
  London SW6 3JD
  (071 371 9717)

THERAPY

Association of Independent Psychotherapists,
  PO Box 1194,
  London N6 5PW
  (071 266 3340)
  Individual therapy from £12 to £30 per hour.
  Also available: couples' counselling.

British Association for Counselling,
  1 Regent Place,
  Rugby,
  Warwickshire CV21 2PJ
  (0788 578328)
  Main umbrella organisation for counselling in Britain with recognised code of ethics. For free local information, phone, or write with A5-sized SAE.

Westminster Pastoral Foundation,
  23 Kensington Square,
  London W8 5HN
  (071 937 6956)
  Individual, group and family therapy in forty-eight affiliated centres across England, Scotland and Wales. Sliding-scale fees.

ADVISORY SERVICES

National Association for Premenstrual Syndrome,
  PO Box 72,
  Sevenoaks,
  Kent TN13 1XQ
  Information line: 0732 741709

PMS Help,
  PO Box 160,
  St Albans,
  Herts AL1 4UQ

The Women's Nutritional Advisory Service,
  PO Box 268,
  Lewes BN7 2QN
  (0732 741709)

British Acupuncture Accreditation Board,
   179 Gloucester Place,
   London NW1 6DX
   (071 724 5330)

British Homeopathic Association,
   27a Devonshire Street,
   London W1N 1RJ
   (071 935 2163)
   Send SAE for list of practitioners.

The Association of Reflexologists,
   110 John Silkin Lane,
   London SE8 5BE
   (071 237 6523)

British Reflexology Association,
   Monks Orchard,
   Whitbourne,
   Worcester WR6 5RB

FAMILY PLANNING AND WELL WOMAN CLINICS

These clinics can provide advice and treatment for PMS and other women's health problems. For your nearest clinic, look in your local telephone directory.

Bibliography

Birke, Linda and Gardner, Katy, *Why Suffer? Periods and Their Problems*, London, Virago, 1984

Duckworth, Helen, *Premenstrual Syndrome: Your Options*, Dublin, Attic Press, 1989

Eichenbaum, Luise and Orbach, Susie, *What Do Women Want?*, London, Fontana, 1984

Fletcher, Eileen, *The Optimum Health Guide: For the Whole of Life*, London, Hodder and Stoughton, 1993

Graham, Judy, *Evening Primrose Oil*, London, Thorsons, 1984

Harrison, Dr Michelle, *Self-Help with PMS*, London, Optima, 1987

Hay, Louise L., *You Can Heal Your Life*, London, Eden Grove Editions, 1984

King, Lesley and Lawrence, Bob, *Luna – a Proving*, Helios Homoeopathic Pharmacy, 97 Camden Road, Tunbridge Wells, Kent TN12 2QR, 1993

Kingston, Beryl, *Lifting the Curse: How to Relieve Painful Periods*, London, Sheldon Press, 1984

Litvinoff, Sarah, *The Relate Guide to Better Relationships*, London, Ebury Press, 1991

Mitchell, Laura, *Simple Relaxation: The Mitchell Method for Easing Tension*, London, John Murray, 1987

Skynner, Robin and Cleese, John, *Families and how to survive them*, London, Methuen, 1983

Stewart, Maryon, *Beat PMT Through Diet*, London, Ebury Press, 1990

Aromatherapy for the Family, London, Wigmore Publications, 1993

Homoepathy for the Family, London, Wigmore Publications, 1991

Vitamins and Minerals, London, Holland and Barrett, 1986

Index

Headline Health Kicks

Positive and practical advice to relieve persistent health problems.
Titles available include:

THE PRIME OF YOUR LIFE
Self help during menopause   Pamela Armstrong   £5.99   ☐

STOP COUNTING SHEEP
Self help for insomnia sufferers   Dr Paul Clayton   £5.99   ☐

AM I A MONSTER, OR IS THIS PMS?
Self help for PMS sufferers   Louise Roddon   £5.99   ☐

GET UP AND GO!
Self help for fatigue sufferers   Anne Woodham   £5.99   ☐

You can kick that problem!

All Headline books are available at your local bookshop or newsagent, or can be ordered direct from the publisher. Just tick the titles you want and fill in the form below. Prices and availability subject to change without notice.

Headline Book Publishing Ltd, Cash Sales Department, Bookpoint, 39 Milton Park, Abingdon, OXON, OX14 4TD, UK. If you have a credit card you may order by telephone – 0235 831700.

Please enclose a cheque or postal order made payable to Bookpoint Ltd to the value of the cover price and allow the following for postage and packing:

UK & BFPO: £1.00 for the first book, 50p for the second book and 30p for each additional book ordered up to a maximum charge of £3.00.

OVERSEAS & EIRE: £2.00 for the first book, £1.00 for the second book and 50p for each additional book.

Name...

Address...

....

....

If you would prefer to pay by credit card, please complete:
Please debit my Visa/Access/Diner's Card/American Express (delete as applicable) card no:

☐☐☐☐☐☐☐☐☐☐☐☐☐☐☐☐☐☐

Signature...   Expiry date...................